T0186657

Psychosocial Assessment in Terminal Care

Psychosocial Assessment in Terminal Care

David M. Dush
Barrie R. Cassileth and Dennis C. Turk
Editors

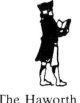

The Haworth Press
New York • London

Psychosocial Assessment in Terminal Care has also been published as *The Hospice Journal: Physical, Psychosocial, and Pastoral Care of the Dying,* Volume 2, Number 3, Fall 1986.

The Haworth Press, Inc., 12 West 32 Street, New York, NY 10001
EUROSPAN/Haworth, 3 Henrietta Street, London, WC2E 8LU England

Library of Congress Cataloging-in-Publication Data

Psychosocial assessment in terminal care.
    "Has also been published as the Hospice journal, volume 2, number 3, fall 1986"—T.p. verso.
    Includes bibliographies.
    1. Terminal care—Psychological aspects. 2. Terminal care—Social aspects. 3. Terminally ill—Testing.
I. Dush, David M. II. Cassileth, Barrie R. III. Turk, Dennis C. [DNLM: 1. Adaptation, Psychological.
2. Hospices. 3. Social Adjustment. 4. Terminal Care—psychology. W1 H069H v.2 no.3 / WB 310 P974]
R726.8.P78   1986   616'.029'019   86-22801
ISBN 0-86656-461-6

Psychosocial Assessment in Terminal Care

The Hospice Journal
Volume 2, Number 3

CONTENTS

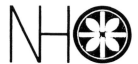

National Hospice Organization

The National Hospice Organization was created to promote and maintain quality care for the terminally ill and their families. Formally established in 1978, NHO is an independent, non-profit, membership association devoted exclusively to hospice.

NATIONAL HOSPICE ORGANIZATION BOARD OF DIRECTORS

FROM THE EDITORS

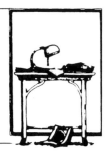

We are pleased to introduce this special collection of papers on psychosocial assessment and measurement. Psychosocial care is, by definition, one of the cornerstones of hospice and palliative terminal care. Its intended outcomes are difficult to operationalize, observe, or measure. Yet, accountability, individualization of psychosocial care, and evaluation of the effectiveness of psychosocial interventions rest upon the ability of clinicians and researchers to accurately assess and track psychosocial functioning and experiences of patients and their families.

There is a vast body of literature available on psychological assessment and measurement; very little has yet been written that addresses the special concerns intrinsic to assessment of the terminally ill and their families. The present collection of papers begins to elucidate the range of these special concerns, and the depth of their complexity. Each paper examines specific methodological considerations in terminal care. Additionally, several important content areas are discussed at length: assessment of pain, assessment of distress in children, evaluation of cognitive functioning, and measurement of patient and family satisfaction.

Not all content areas relevant to psychosocial care are represented, nor are all methodological topics. This collection

1

does provide a beginning, however, and a focus for the important research that lies ahead.

David M. Dush, PhD
Barrie R. Cassileth, PhD
Dennis C. Turk, PhD
Editors

Lessons From Hospice Evaluations

Robert L. Kane

The hospice movement was imported to North America with
great enthusiasm. The initial reports of the pioneering work at
St. Christopher's in London and the Royal Victoria Palliative
Care Unit at Montreal encouraged American importers to
make extravagant promises. Some of the initial enthusiasm for
this concept might be explained by the hyperbole often associated with the introduction of new movements and the need to
sell innovative concepts by promising dramatic effects. At the
same time, it is also important to recognize that the hospice
movement was more than an innovation in care delivery; it was
part of the general reformation in the way we approach the
care of dying persons. It represented a refutation of the cold,
professional, highly technical and austere care typified by the
modern scientific hospital. The hospice promised a humaniza-
tion with subsequent improvements in the way individuals
faced the last weeks and months of their lives.

Ironically, hospice also represented its *own* technology. It
was particularly intent on developing new methods on pain
control and on using psychoactive medications as minimally as
possible to avoid impairing cognitive function while reducing
psychological stress by environmental manipulations. Promised outcomes then generally focused around issues of improved pain management and subsequent reduction in pain
and discomfort, a reduction in the side effects of drug therapy
(particularly narcotics and psychoactive drugs), improvement
in affect and greater satisfaction. Moreover, the beneficiaries
of hospice care were not only the dying individuals, but their
families as well. Support provided to families, both directly
and indirectly, during the course of the death of the patient
and subsequently during bereavement was expected to relieve

Robert L. Kane, MD, is the Dean of the School of Public Health, University of
Minnesota, Box 197 Mayo, 420 Delaware Street S. E., Minneapolis, MN 55455.

3

some of the stress around the dying process and the adverse consequences of bereavement. All of this was to be done for a price lower than traditional hospital-based care.

It is worthwhile to examine the experiences of the major evaluations of hospice efforts to appreciate the controversies that arose when the results were made public and to explore some of the generic issues which confront these evaluations and others along similar lines. In general, the findings of the two major hospice evaluation studies to date were rather consistent. They basically reported that hospice care was not generally better than conventional care, but it was no worse. Each of the two major studies—the National Hospice Study and the UCLA randomized controlled trial—found some instances in which hospice care was better than the control group, but in most of the areas examined there was no difference. Where there were differences, they tended to be around the levels of satisfaction, expressed by patients or their families; differences did not occur around pain control, affect, or symptoms. (Greer, Mor, Morris, Sherwood, Kidder, & Birnbaum, in press; Kane, Bergstein, Wales, & Rothberg, 1985a; Kane, Klein, Bergstein, & Rothberg, in press; Kane, Klein, Bergstein, Rothberg, & Wales, 1985b; Kane, Wales, Bergstein et al., 1984). The National Hospice Study found that the cost of home-based hospice care was cheaper than conventional care (Birnbaum & Kidder, 1984). The UCLA study, which employed largely a hospital-based model of hospice care, found no difference in the cost of care (Kane et al., 1984).

In looking at the issue of evaluating hospice care, it seems most appropriate to focus on the question of effectiveness. Although the pressures for policy-relevant information call for *cost*-effectiveness data, it is important first to establish whether the new therapy is indeed effective. This may be better termed a test of efficacy. Under the conditions of such testing, one wants to examine the best models of care available. If the efficacy can be established, then one can go on to ask questions about how one can maintain the performance level while reducing the cost. Experience with hospice care has shown that much of the cost question is going to be established by external events at any rate. Certainly once hospices became covered as a Medicare benefit, the question quickly became how much care could one provide for the price being paid. Fortunately, the two major studies being discussed here were carried out without active constraints imposed by cost restrictions.

The design of any evaluation poses problems. In the case of the hospice, some specific issues need to be considered. The randomized controlled trial is generally acknowledged as the strongest possible experimental design to test a new innovation. However, the very process of random assignment imposes certain constraints. Although all participants have been queried about their willingness to participate in the experiment and to receive the therapy if proffered, the very heart of the random allocation denies the individual subject the choice in seeking the therapy or not. From the standpoint of policy relevant information, one might be more interested in the results of self-selection. Does the treatment modality work for those who want it? In practical application they will be the ones who use it. On the one hand, such self-selection represents a strong bias; on the other, if the question is re-posed to compare those who specifically select a treatment against those who do not, a more policy relevant approach may be pursued. In the best of all possible worlds, one would want to look at some combination of information based on such self-selection and a parallel design in which the true efficacy of the intervention is tested through a randomized controlled trial. In effect, we have the combination of this information available with regard to hospice care. The UCLA study is a randomized trial. As such it is limited to a single site and a single modality of care. The national study had to use a quasi-experimental design to compare two types of hospice care (home care and hospital-based care) with conventional care in several locations.

Both the National Hospice Study and the UCLA study spent extensive periods in meeting with advocates of the hospice movement to establish the criteria for the evaluation (Greer et al., 1983; Wales et al., 1983). All of the data parameters were developed in response to specific criteria identified by professionals involved in hospice care. An issue quickly arises as to whether such measures should be developed specifically for the hospice program or whether one should seek to adapt wherever possible extant measures with established validity and wider applicability than simply a hospice program. From the standpoint of establishing policy relevant information, the latter course is generally more desirable. The use of widely applied measures allows for more generalizability and easier comparisons with other investigations along similar or related lines. However, the failure to find differences will readily lead to a concern about the sensitivity and appropriateness of the measures. Although it is crucial that outcomes not be unspecified, it is dangerous to insist on custom-made measures to detect differences (McCuster, 1984). In many instances the measures designed to catch the nuance of the intervention may introduce their own bias. For most policy purposes, the effects sought should be gross enough to permit easy detection. Differences on a scale score are not as impressive as a reduction in days lost from work, for example.

A number of specific methodologic problems were posed by the hospice studies. One of the most difficult was the source of information. Clearly the usual problems of respondent and burden are magnified in a situation where one is dealing with dying individuals. From an ethical standpoint, one is concerned about being overly voyeuristic and intrusive. From a practical standpoint any of the subjects may quickly reach a stage where they can no longer tolerate the burden of a lengthy questionnaire, if they can respond at all. At the same time, one must question the validity of information derived from a second party. It seems much less satisfactory to try to obtain information about another individual's pain, their affect, or their satisfaction. The area of measuring pain poses the most difficult problems in any event. We lack any real ways to validate such measures and for the most part do not even have an adequate vocabulary to describe or to quantify these feelings in any very reliable manner.

One concern sometimes expressed about the evaluation process is the extension of the Heisenberg Principle. The frequent contacts with control group members in order to obtain comparable measures on the effect of the intervention (or lack thereof) may in and of itself become an intervention with therapeutic potential. Particularly in a situation like hospice care where much of the support being offered is in the form of general social support, the concerned interviewer may represent a therapist. Here we are caught in a familiar paradox.

On the one hand we are arguing that we are offering a new service that is powerful and distinct. On the other hand, we have the suggestion that the differences in impact created by the service are so vulnerable that they can be offset by periodic contacts with the control population. If indeed the service is that fragile, one must question its importance. A similar argument is often made for the indirect effects of hospice care on the surrounding therapeutic community. Concerns are expressed about the probabilities of the hospice concept diffusing to change the behaviors of conventional therapists. While one would certainly want to acknowledge the contribution of the hospice movement as part of the general movement in thanatology, again one must note that if it were that easy to change the behavior of conventional care givers, the investment in hospice care would probably not be necessary.

The hospice evaluations were careful to measure outcomes along a variety of dimensions, including pain control, affect, and satisfaction. One might well ask whether any differences in areas other than satisfaction were really necessary. If indeed we are looking at a service provided to terminally ill individuals, is it not sufficient that they experience a more satisfactory service during their last days (Rainey, Crane, Breslow, & Granz, 1984)? This question raises a basic dilemma for policy makers. In general we have been uncomfortable using satisfaction as a sufficient condition for outcomes of service. We have been led to expect differences in other more professionally recognized parameters. Partly because we fear the placebo effect of a new service, particularly one that has been introduced with great fanfare, and partly because we have been trained to look for more empirically verifiable measures of impact, we are generally dissatisfied with satisfaction as the only measure of success. One points quickly to experience with cancer patients and laetrile as an example of false therapy. However, in the case of hospice, the therapy is not intended to delay mortality, but simply to improve the quality of the available time.

We are left then with a body of information which suggests that hospice care does provide an appropriate alternative form of therapy for terminally ill persons, particularly those who prefer that mode of care. Ironically, were the hospice advocates to abandon some of their more extravagant claims, there would be no controversy about the role of hospice as a legitimate form of therapy. Evaluation concerns could then shift to a second tier of questions such as for whom is hospice therapy most effective and what variations in hospice form might be best matched to each of the various potential target groups. There remain interesting questions about just what constitutes a hospice. Is it the presence of certain positive features or the absence of negative ones? However, the hospice orthodoxy has not yet come to terms with the consistency of the evaluation results. There remains discomfort with the confrontation of an attractive idea with empirical data. This apparent conflict is reminiscent of similar difficulties when claims for unconventional therapies designed to develop positive affects for an illness were shown to be without empirical basis when dying patients were actually studied (Cassileth et al., 1984).

REFERENCES

Birnbaum, H. G., & Kidder, D. (1984). What does hospice cost? *American Journal of Public Health, 74,* 689–697.

Cassileth, B. R., Lusk, E. J., Matazzo, I., Thompson, C. J., Brown, L. L., Cross, P. A., & Tenaglia, A. N. (1984). Psychosocial status in chronic illness: A comparative analysis of six diagnostic groups. *New England Journal of Medicine, 311,* 506–511.

Greer, D. S., Mor, V., Morris, J. N., Sherwood, S., Kidder, D., & Birnbaum, H. (in press). An alternative in terminal care: Results of the National Hospice Study. *Journal of Chronic Diseases.*

Greer, D. S., Mor, V., Sherwood, S., et al. (1983). National Hospice Analysis Plans. *Journal of Chronic Diseases, 36,* 737–780.

Kane, R. L., Bernstein, L., Wales, J., & Rothberg, R. (1985a). Hospice effectiveness in controlling pain. *Journal of the American Medical Association, 253,* 2683–2686.

Kane, R. L., Klein, S. J., Bernstein, L., & Rothberg, R. (in press). The role of hospice in reducing the impact of bereavement. *Journal of Chronic Diseases.*

Kane, R. L., Klein, S. J., Bernstein, L., Rothberg, R., & Wales, J. (1985b). Hospice role in alleviating the emotional stress of terminal patients and their families. *Medical Care, 23,* 189–197.

Kane, R. L., Wales, J., Bernstein, L., et al. (1984). A randomized controlled trial of hospice care. *Lancet, 1,* 890–894.

McCuster, J. (1984). Development of scales to measure satisfaction in preferences regarding long-term and terminal care. *Medical Care, 22,* 476–492.

Rainey, L. C., Crane, L. A., Breslow, D. M., & Ganz, P. A. (1984). Cancer patient's attitude toward hospice services. *CA/A Cancer Journal for Clinicians, 34,* 191–201.

Wales, J., Kane, R. L., Robbins, S., et al. (1983). The UCLA Hospice Evaluation Study: Methodology and instrumentation. *Medical Care, 21,* 734–744.

Lessons From Hospice Evaluations: Counterpoint

John J. Mahoney

In this edition of *The Hospice Journal* the reader will find an article, "Lessons From Hospice Evaluations" by Robert L. Kane, M.D. Dr. Kane is a respected scientist and researcher, currently the Dean of the School of Public Health at the University of Minnesota. In my view, however, Dr. Kane has left the role of researcher and taken on the mantle of social commentator in this article. Consequently, I offer this counterpoint to his arguments.

Kane's article is based on test results generated from the Brown University Study (The National Hospice Study) and a study conducted by Dr. Kane at the UCLA Veterans Administration Hospital. Dr. Kane uses these results to support his hypothesis that while hospice care does provide an appropriate alternative form of therapy for terminally ill persons, it is, comparatively speaking, no better or worse than conventional care.

The Final Report of the National Hospice Study has not been released by the Health Care Financing Administration; however, in 1984 Dr. Barrie Cassileth, then Chairman of the NHO Research and Evaluation Committee, made the following observations regarding the "quality of life" results produced in the preliminary Brown University report:[1]

A methodologic problem with the Brown University study was its manner of assessing patients' quality of life. It would have been difficult, as the Brown report noted, for some terminally-ill patients to complete questionnaires. Most quality of life questionnaires available at the time of their study were indeed physically and men-

John J. Mahoney is the President of the National Hospice Organization, 1901 North Fort Myer Drive, Suite 307, Arlington, VA 22209.

tally taxing. Brown University used the next best device then available: caregiving and assessment with a questionnaire based on Spitzer's Quality of Life Index.

The difficulty with caregiver assessment is twofold. First, quality of life is extremely subjective and personal. No one but the individual can truly assess the quality of his own life. If there were such a thing as "objective" quality of life, we would not have suicides among young, healthy, attractive people, nor would there be so few suicides among seriously disabled or fatally-ill patients, whose "objective" quality of life is extremely poor. Therefore, assessment of one person's quality of life by another produces indirect information and questionable results.

The second difficulty with caregiver assessment is that caregivers may sense the patient's quality of life to be a reflection of the effectiveness of their own caregiving. Caring families could not emotionally sustain the idea that their efforts were ineffective, resulting in poor quality of life for the patient. Positive caregiver assessment reflects the caregiver's own experience, which is very important as such. Here, it is tantamount to saying: "I have done my best; we have found the best place and the best care for our loved one."

Some of these points pertain as well to the issue of patient satisfaction. Hospice and non-hospice patients in the Brown University study were found to be equally satisfied with their care. Patients in any setting tend to express satisfaction with care that they selected and on which they are dependent during a critical and vulnerable time in their lives. Expressing dissatisfaction with care would be equivalent to feeling that one made a bad choice and is incapable of altering the situation, a position of emotional discomfort that patients, and the rest of us, tend to avoid. A fundamental psychological phenomenon or facet of human nature is our tendency to feel very positive about major decisions once we have made them.

Finally, quality of life probably is closely related to disease or clinical status. We do not know from the Brown

University Study whether patients in home-based hospice programs were similar in terms of disease status to patients in hospital-based programs. It is possible that a process of self-selection occurred here, with sicker patients going to hospital-based hospice programs than to home-based programs.

An additional problem is one that is intrinsic to many studies of human beings. When a person or a program knows that it is part of a study, that very knowledge can alter its behavior or quality. We do not know the extent to which programs of the same type were similar to one another, nor do we know whether different types of programs grew to become similar to one another as a function of being studied.

We must view the quality of life results with caution, understanding that not patients, but others assessed patients' quality of life, that "satisfaction" with care is difficult to measure meaningfully, and that these issues generally are fraught with numerous influencing variables and therefore extremely difficult to assess.[2]

Also, as part of the same NHO Monograph, Dr. Cassileth wrote the following regarding Dr. Kane's conclusion (in the UCLA study) that hospice care does not seem to make a qualitative difference:

Hospice patients in this study spent about as many days in the hospital (51 days) as did non-hospice patients (48 days). However, this is an example of how data can be misleading and interpreted in more than one way. The UCLA article compared the average number of inpatient days for hospice versus non-hospice patients, rather than the average proportion or percent of inpatient days, and it did not include nursing home days in the inpatient calculation. Using information given in the (study), and including nursing home days as inpatient days, hospice patients spent an average of 52 days as inpatients (54% of their time), and non-hospice patients spent an average of 59 days as inpatients (61% of their time). Looking at these same figures from the "days at home" point of view, hospice patients spent 46% of their time at home, while non-hospice patients spent 39% of their time at home. This meaningful difference was not discussed in the article.

Similarly, information about major treatment procedures is reported in a way that makes it difficult to evaluate the impact of hospice. The average number of procedures per patient (less than one for each hospice as well as non-hospice patient) is reported. However, we are not told whether hospice patients received chemotherapy, radiation therapy, or surgery when they were in the hospice inpatient unit or when they were cared for elsewhere in the hospital. (Hospital patients spent an average of 29 days on the hospice unit, 13 days on general medical floors, and 8 days in "intermediate care." That is, only slightly over half of hospice patients' inpatient time was spent on the hospice unit.) It is possible that palliative treatment was needed and ordered appropriately by hospice staff; it is possible alternatively that these procedures were ordered by conventional staff during patients' stays in conventional areas of the hospital. This is not discussed, nor is there mention of the fact that palliative treatment techniques may be a needed and appropriate component of hospice care.

The (study's) conclusion that "Intensive hospice care did not yield the expected benefits in pain or symptom relief or in alleviation of psychological distress . . ." is arguable on two counts. First, the hospice patients in this study did not receive "intensive" hospice care. They received a mix of hospice and conventional care. Second, benefits in pain, symptom relief, and psychological distress occurred in the best of ways: even patients under conventional care benefited from the skills that their conventional caregivers learned from hospice staff.

There is a methodologic concern with regard to quality of life results. Quality of life was measured in patients who were at different points in time vis à vis proximity to death. That is, patients who were very sick and near to death, and patients who were less sick and much further from death, were mixed together to obtain average quality of life data. This is a confounding feature that should be kept in mind when evaluating these results.

In addition, remember that the patient sample in this study was comprised of patients at a Veterans' Administration hospital. Almost all patients were male, and neither patients nor their families are representative sociodemographically of the general population. Finally, the home care component of the UCLA study is not addressed, and we do not know how this important hospice feature (or its absence) influenced study results.[2]

In addition, in the September 1985 issue of *Oncology Times* (Vol. VII, No. 9, pp. 2, 14), Dr. Yale Penzell, a hospice physician in the UCLA Veterans Administration Hospice (the site of Dr. Kane's study) wrote the following regarding Dr. Kane's findings:

As the Kane study points out, the Hospice Program at the VA West Los Angeles Medical Center consists of three components: Consultation, Home Care, and the Hospice Inpatient Unit. In creating the "hospice (experimental)" group that purports to represent a typical hospice sampling, the researchers failed to make clear that, to a great degree, the Hospice physician *does not* (author's italics) prescribe medications for pain and symptom control for a large percentage of that group, i.e., the Consultation and Home Care patients.

The main function of the Home Care component is to provide nursing care, psychological support, and social services and to act as a liaison between the patients and various hospital specialty clinics whose physicians are in charge of their care. Only in a small percentage of cases (when the patient has no primary physician or is housed on the Hospice Inpatient Unit) are the medications for pain and symptom control ever prescribed by the Hospice physician. Most of the Home Care and Consultation patients in the study were receiving such "traditional" care as radiation treatment, chemotherapy, and surgery, and undergoing diagnostic tests under treatment plans designed and implemented by physicians in the outpatient clinics or on other wards in the hospital.

All of the 137 "hospice (experimental)" group were initially assigned to the Consultation Service. The Hospice Consultation Team saw the patient, reviewed his chart, and decided whether to admit him to the Home Care program, the Inpatient Unit, or to follow him on Consultation. Thirty-seven of these patients remained on other wards throughout the duration of the study and were never under the direct care of the Hospice physician, still, these Consultation patients were considered "hospice" patients for the purposes of the study.

Only 40 of the 137 "hospice" patients were under the direct orders of the Hospice physician more than 50% of the time, and only 24 of these patients were under the care of the Hospice physician more than 75% of the time.

With its focus on pain and symptom control, and emotional and psychological support, hospice care has helped to ease both the physical and psychological pain of dying for the terminally ill and their families. This flawed study does a great disservice to the hospice movement and to the people who might yet benefit from the skilled, humane care hospice provides.[3]

A final point regarding Dr. Kane's conclusions is drawn from his own article.[4] Dr. Kane states that in evaluating hospice care it seems most appropriate to focus on the question of effectiveness. And, in order to compare the effectiveness of hospice care it is necessary to use widely applied measures allowing far more generalizability and easier comparison.

Pain control is arguably one of the most important questions regarding the quality of life in a terminally ill person and the effectiveness of hospice care. Dr. Kane's article clearly states:

The area of measuring pain poses the most difficult problem in any event. We lack real ways to validate such measures and for the most part do not even have an adequate vocabulary to describe or to quantify these feelings in any very reliable manner.[4]

To state that it is difficult, if not impossible, to adequately measure and compare one of the most important aspects of hospice care, and then to conclude that hospice care really does not make much difference appears to be an editorial conclusion of Dr. Kane's, not supportable by his research at UCLA or Brown University's "National Hospice Study."

Hospice care, quite honestly, is probably not the panacea that some in the hospice community would insist it is. However, neither science nor the legitimate claims of hospice proponents are served by the sweeping conclusions of Dr. Kane's articles in light of closer examination of the studies used to support those conclusions.

REFERENCES

1. Greer DS, Mor U, Birnbaum H, Sherwood S, Morris NJ. National hospice study preliminary final report (extended executive summary). Providence: Brown University, 1983.

2. Cassileth BR. Major Hospice Research Projects Review and Evaluation Arlington: National Hospice Organization, 1984.

3. Penzel Y. Letter to the Editor, *Oncology Times,* Vol. VII, No. 9, 1985.

4. Kane R.L. Lessons From Hospice Evaluations, *The Hospice Journal,* this issue.

Assessing Patient Outcomes in Hospice: What to Measure?

Vincent Mor

INTRODUCTION

The hospice philosophy states that "hospice exists to provide support and care for patients . . . so that they might live as fully and comfortably as possible" (NHO, 1979). Focus on the psychosocial status of hospice patients is grounded in this philosophy and reflects the emphasis that hospice places upon meeting the needs of the whole person. Clearly, measures of the outcomes hospice patients experience under the care of a hospice should reflect the goals and values of the care model if we are to adequately monitor whether these goals are met. In conceiving of how to measure patient outcomes, it is critical to fully examine the implications of alternate measurement approaches.

The current paper briefly examines existing literature related to measuring the principal hospice goals and identifies issues and complications associated with measuring these constructs. Drawing upon data obtained as part of the National Hospice Study (NHS), the fit between various approaches to measuring patients' psychosocial status, quality of life, and the physical conditions of terminal cancer patients are examined.

A Review of Measurement Issues

Using basic notions of measurement validity and reliability as a point of departure, this section reviews a series of compli-

This work was supported in part by DHHS/HCFA Grant #99-P-97793, and grants from the Robert Wood Johnson Foundation and the John A. Hartford Foundation. Vincent Mor, PhD, is an associate professor, Department of Community Health, Brown University, and Director, Center for Health Care Research, Brown University, Box G, Providence, RI 02912.

cations inherent in measuring the psychosocial status of terminally ill cancer patients. The issues addressed are; (1) using
scales standardized on other populations, (2) measuring different dimensions of quality of life, (3) patient non-response,
(4) appropriate sources of data when the patient is non-re-
sponsive, and (5) appropriateness of the measure to the hospice patient population.

Using standardized scales that have not been tested for the
specific population in question can, under some circumstances, yield highly misleading results (Nunnally, 1967). For
example, the use of standardized indices of depression that
rely heavily on the contribution of somatic symptoms in
evaluating the level of depression consistently overestimate
depression in medically ill samples such as the terminally ill
cancer patient (Craig and Abeloff, 1974; Derogatis et al.,
1983; Plumb and Holland, 1977). Derogatis and his colleagues
identified only 6% of a random sample of cancer patients as
having a DSM-III diagnosis of major depression. On the
other hand, Peck maintains that nearly 75% of hospital patients have the syndrome of clinical depression (1972). Craig
and Abeloff (1974) noted that the heterogeneity of samples
examined and the variability in instruments and approaches
used to ascertain the presence of depression all contributed to
the obvious confusion about the prevalence of depression
among cancer patients.

The importance of disentangling the somatic from the non-
somatic when assessing terminal cancer patients' psychosocial
status is borne out by Plumb and Holland's paper (1977).
They separated the physical and non-physical components of
the Beck Depression Inventory and found that while cancer
patients resembled persons who had attempted suicide on the
physical dimensions of depression, they resembled healthy
next of kin on the non-physical components. Since most depression scales completed either by raters or via self-report
were designed for use in a psychiatric population which does
not have the level of physical illness associated with the terminally ill, particular care must be taken in interpreting results.

Not only is there a conceptual problem associated with
measuring psychosocial status among cancer patients, but the
psychometric properties of scales developed for very different
populations can make their application problematic. For ex-

ample, the Profile of Mood States (POMS), often used in cancer patient populations, was standardized on psychiatric patients (McNair, Lorr, and Droppleman, 1981). Average levels of mood disturbance among cancer patients reported in the literature are almost uniformly lower than those reported by the authors of the tests (Cassileth et al., 1985; Goldberg et al., 1984). While patients with more advanced disease have higher mood disturbance scores, this can be attributed to reduced vigor and energy, both components of the overall score and the depression scale. The relatively high standard deviations observed in cancer patient populations also suggest that there is considerable skew in the distribution of responses, with most respondents reporting little or no mood disturbance on any of the non-somatic dimensions of the scale.

The multidimensional nature of psychosocial status has often been noted (Greer et al., 1983; Linn et al., 1980). While investigators have tended to focus upon the mood state aspects of psychosocial status, factors such as social interaction, contentment, and the absence of pain and distressing symptoms can also be classed as psychosocial status. Spitzer and his colleagues (1981) undertook a cross-national effort to standardize a measure of global quality of life which incorporates physical, social, and psychological dimensions. The qualities identified as being the "kingpins" of quality of life were those chosen by samples of lay and professional persons as essential ingredients to having a high quality of life. This "consensual" approach to validity was also subjected to construct validation by comparing the relative "quality of life" of advanced cancer patients with that of other classes of healthy and impaired adults (Spitzer et al., 1981). Advanced cancer patients were found to have lower quality of life than the other groups. Subsequent analyses of this scale revealed that the quality of life scale was sensitive to the decreases in functioning associated with the approach of death (Morris, Suizza, et al., 1986).

Non-response of patients to psychosocial items can be due to a variety of factors. Loss of cognitive clarity due to brain metastases or medication side effects can alter patients' responses. Missing patient information may often be due to requirements for signed informed consent. Excessive symptoms such as pain, nausea, and shortness of breath can greatly diminish the patients' capacity to undertake the occasionally lengthy process of interviews containing standardized psychological testing. Just as with old age, increased symptomatology may affect concentration, stamina, or response acquiescence (Lawton, Whelihan, and Belsky, 1980). Unfortunately, few researchers publish data about the proportion of subjects able to be tested using particular instruments. Lawton and his colleagues summarized the personality assessment literature as applied to the aged and showed that the shorter the test, the lower the rate of non-complete response. Obviously, one suspects responders to differ substantially from non-responders in terms of performance, mood state, etc., drawing the representativeness of responders into question.

Alternate sources of information when the patient is unable to be interviewed can be caretaking staff, families, or independent observers. Staff members as informants or observers have a vested interest in minimizing the unresolved problems experienced by the patient, especially if they perceive the information to be at all evaluative in nature (Campbell, 1975). Use of trained observers is very costly and presents its own problems with respect to inter-observer reliability (Sechrest, 1985). In addition to the technical problems of data gathering, use of observers requires very careful operational definition of the concepts to be observed. In the case of psychosocial status and mood state, agreement about the definition of the constructs would be even more difficult than agreement about observations of patients' functioning.

Using family members as informants can also be biased. Since families are major providers of care, their assessments of the patients might reflect their own need to minimize the pain and problems the patient experiences. Alternately, they may overestimate the problems the patient experiences because they cannot imagine how they themselves could endure the conditions they see the patient endure. Despite these potential biases, the family caretaker both knows the patient best and is in the best position to comment about the patient's condition since he or she is almost constantly with the patient. As such, this person can presumably observe and report even slight changes in the patient's condition, as evidenced by both verbal and nonverbal attempts that patients make to communicate their needs. Regardless of whether the family member may "accurately" portray the picture of the patient at any point in time, monitoring *changes* in the family member's perspective over time may have validity from a relativistic perspective.

Sufficient data examining the response of cancer patients and their families now exist to surmise that the conditions of the patients' family members and caretakers rise and fall with that of the patient and his disease state (Cassileth et al., 1985; Gotay, 1984). This is quite different from attesting to the validity of the caretaker's reports on the patient's condition. It is, however, consistent with the hospice notion that patients and families should be treated as a unit. If the patient and family are the unit of care and their emotional or psychological states covary over time, then perhaps it is reasonable to allow the family member to serve as a proxy for measuring the patient's condition when it is not possible to do so directly. In the NHS, we found that patients' and their primary care persons' assessment of the pain that they were experiencing were moderately, although not strongly (.43), correlated (Morris, Mor, Goldberg, et al., 1986). Similarly, other patient symptoms assessed by the primary care person were moderately well correlated.

Matching the measure to the population presents a special problem of the patient with advanced cancer. A review of the literature describing hospice patients (Mor, in press) revealed that across nearly 15,000 patients studied, the weighted average length of stay of hospice patients was some 45 days with a median of 30 days. In the NHS, over one-fourth of the 13,374 patients studied were completely incontinent upon admission to hospice, and nearly one-fifth required oxygen (Greer, Mor, and Kastenbaum, in press). These data all point to a highly vulnerable patient, one who frequently cannot be asked questions about his or her condition around the time of hospice admission. Nearly one-quarter of patients die within 10 days of admission, meaning that the amount of time hospice staff have to mount an intensive, personalized psychosocial intervention is extremely limited. For longer stay patients, needs are likely to change as their disease progresses along its inevitable path (Morris, Suizza, et al., 1986). Consequently, since many hospice patients will experience only the advanced terminal phase under hospice care, it is the problems of that phase with which we must reckon in assessing the outcomes of hospice care.

Having raised this series of issues regarding the measurement and choice of psychosocial constructs that are appropriate for hospice, the next section of this paper reviews selected findings of the National Hospice Study in proposing a hierarchy of outcomes to which hospice should attend. The interpretation of the data is not merely relevant to researchers interested in evaluating the outcomes of care at a particular hospice. It is also relevant for hospice staff and administrators as they face difficult choices of resource allocation in the future.

METHODS

Sites and Samples

Data for the current report were assembled on hospice patients selected by predetermined criteria from a population of over 12,000 terminal cancer patients served by 40 hospices distributed nationally. Twenty-six of the hospices received special Medicare demonstration waivers allowing payment for normally non-covered services. Study sites were not randomly selected because the demonstration hospices had been chosen competitively by the Health Care Financing Administration (HCFA) from a pool of 233 applicants; nondemonstration hospices were therefore selected by the evaluators to resemble demonstration sites organizationally. Details regarding the sampling methodology, measures used, and study findings have been presented elsewhere (Greer et al., 1983; Greer et al., 1986; Greer, Mor, and Kastenbaum, in press).

The sample considered in this report consisted of cancer patients and their families served in hospices who consented to participate in a "follow-up" study. Follow-up study eligibility was based upon: (a) cancer confirmed by tissue diagnosis (except for brain and pancreatic cancer); (b) remote metastasis (except for lung, brain, and pancreatic cancer); (c) presence of a primary care person (PCP), generally a family member in the household; (d) age 21 or older; and (e) for CC patients only, a Karnofsky Performance Status (KPS) (Karnofsky et al., 1948) of 50 or less (i.e., requiring assistance in daily activities). These criteria were based upon a review of modal hospice patient characteristics: 90% have cancer, over 95% have a PCP, almost all are over age 21, and over 90% require assistance with personal care at the time of hospice admission.

A total of 1,457 patients (833 hospital based, 624 home care hospice based) were included in the follow-up sample. Trained and tested interviewers assessed patient eligibility from available records. The refusal rate of patients and PCPs (both had to give written consent) was 3.4% in hospice; dropout among those signing consent forms was 4.4%. Only patients who died during the study period were included in the final analytic samples since outcomes were assessed in relation to proximity to death.

Data Gathering Methods

Personal interviews with the patient and PCP were conducted at study entry. A first follow-up contact occurred 7 days later and was repeated every 14 days thereafter until the patient's death. In addition to the patient interviews, at each contact, the PCP (a) provided data on his or her own condition and attitudes, (b) presented a record of all health services utilized by the patient, and (c) reported on the patient's condition. Information on primary site, histology, metastases, date of disease onset, and prior treatment was obtained from medical records.

Patient Outcome Variables

Measures were adapted or developed to evaluate the impact of hospice. Multiple domains and measures were used, many of which were based upon established scales (Karnofsky et al., 1948; McNair, Lorr, and Droppleman, 1981; Melzack, 1975; Oleson and Bresler, 1979; Spitzer et al., 1981; Wolf et al., 1978). Patient outcome measures were frequently based upon PCP reports since most of the patients could not be interviewed in the weeks just prior to death.

Measures of patient outcome were relatively stable until 5 weeks prior to death (Morris, Suizza, et al., 1986). In addition to analyzing patient changes prospectively from admission date, outcome measures from both patients and PCP were analyzed in relation to date of death. The last measure occurred, on average, 7 days before death. The penultimate measure occurred approximately 21 days pre-death. There were no significant differences among settings in terms of the timing of measurements.

Three sets of measures were employed, each of which was examined for sensitivity to change as patients deteriorated. First, measures of patient *self-reported mood* state were developed—one based upon a subset of the depression scale of the Profile of Mood States (POMS), and another based upon a subset of the Rosenberg Self-Esteem Scale (Rosenberg, 1973). These data were only available when the patient was able to respond to the interview independently. Analyses of summary scales of both measures reveal each to have acceptable levels of reliability (greater than .7). The second set of measures relate to *patient functioning,* as measured by the Karnofsky Performance Status (KPS) index (Karnofsky et al., 1948) and by a modified version of the Spitzer Quality of Life Index (QLI) (Morris, Suizza, et. al., 1986; Spitzer et al., 1981). The KPS was rated by trained, nonmedical interviewers with demonstrated inter-rater reliability. The QLI was recorded by the patient's primary care person (PCP) at each interview. Both measures were correlated and strongly related to patient survival in this population (Mor et al., 1984). The final set of measures reflected a combination of patient and primary care person input pertaining to the presence of symptoms ranging from pain to nausea to difficulty eating. The prevalence of selected symptoms was found to increase as the patient approached death, as would be expected clinically.

FINDINGS

Sample Description

The sample included in these analyses consisted of 1,457 hospice patients with an average age of 68: 41% female, 62% married, and 95% white. Only a small minority of patients lived alone (7.6% among home care hospice patients and

16.1% among hospital based patients). Per study requirements, all patients had a primary care person, most often a
spouse or child (83%) averaging 58 years of age. Forty-three
percent of study patients were served by hospices with their
own beds, and the average length of stay for all patients was
54 days. At the point of entry into hospice, patients were
fairly disabled, with an average Karnofsky Performance Status score of 36 out of 100 (Karnofsky, 1948). Underrepre-
sented in this sample from the population of all hospice patients are those who die very quickly (within a few days) after
admission, and this group may represent as much as 10% of
the hospice population. This underrepresentation should be
kept in mind in interpreting the present findings.

Pattern of Patient Deterioration

Figure 1 presents a backdrop to our examination of reported mood state and quality of life among terminal cancer
patients served in hospice. Over the last 35 days of life, a
period which typically encompasses over half of the length of
stay, we observed an inexorable decline in performance status
and an increase in the number of symptoms experienced.
Both measures were reported by either trained observers or
the PCP. The pattern of decline is consistent with our clinical
observations of similar patients. Within one week of death,
the KPS score is typically around 25, and over half of the
patients are in the moribund or very sick categories.

By the last measure prior to death, the average number (of
a possible 10) symptoms assessed was 5.5, up from 4.4 at
around 35 days prior to death. Most of the increase is attri-
butable to an increasing likelihood of patients to experience
shortness of breath, and trouble swallowing and eating. Any
of these symptoms can make it more difficult to respond to
interview questions. Indeed, the proportion of patients able
to comment upon their own experience of symptom severity
decreased rapidly as death approached. At the last interview
prior to death, only 35.8% of patients seen were able to
answer questions about the severity of their pain, a coverage
priority item for interviewers. At the previous interview, approximately 3 weeks prior to death, 61% of patients responded to the question.

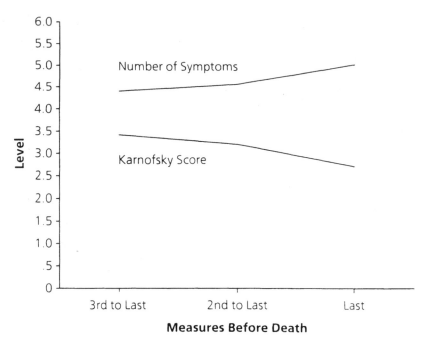

Figure 1

Pattern of Deterioration

Concurrent with physical deterioration and symptoms was a progressive increase in cognitive impairment. By the last week of life, some 20% of patients were unconscious, confused, or completely incapacitated, and only 35% were reported to have their full range of mental capacities. Among patients interviewed within only a few days of death, the proportion unconscious was even higher. These factors combine to make it exceedingly difficult to measure the patient's experience using traditional direct interview techniques at the advanced terminal stage.

Measuring Mood State

The two measures of mood state employed in the NHS were short subsets of existing standardized scales. The subset items were selected on the basis of a careful review of the literature. Components of existing scales that had been used before with cancer patients and found to be sensitive to change and intervention were examined (Greer et al., 1983). Both scales selected were found to be reliable and without excessive skewness or restriction of variance.

Table 1 presents the scale averages for the first 7 interviews. Additionally, the percentage of patients responding at each interview is given in terms of the total sample and as a percent of those still living at any given timeframe. There was virtually no change in the level of depression or self-esteem. The number of responders, however, changed from interview to interview. Therefore, we examined averages among patients responding to at least the first 5 interviews. Again, no significant change emerged.

The major cause of sample attrition was death. Twenty percent of the sample had only an initial interview. Over 40% of the sample were not interviewed a third time, which would have occurred approximately 21 to 25 days after hospice admission. Among the increasingly small group of patients interviewed repeatedly, only half responded to the self-report mood state items. Not only did it become increasingly difficult to contact and see the patient (if still alive), but it was increasingly rare to find the patient capable of responding to the

Table 1

Average Psychosocial Test Scores and

Percentage of Responders at Each Interview Contact

	POMS – Depression	Self- Esteem	Percent of Initial Sample Not Responding	Percent of Living Patients Responding
First Interview	21.9	11.1	40.7	60.3
Second Interview	21.4	11.1	58.7	51.3
Third Interview	22.1	10.7	71.3	48.2
Fourth Interview	22.6	10.8	78.9	50.0
Fifth Interview	22.2	10.6	84.7	47.6
Sixth Interview	22.4	10.3	88.7	45.9
Seventh Interview	21.6	10.7	91.4	44.2

mood state scales. Table 2 supports this observation. The average KPS score of patients who didn't complete the mood state items was consistently significantly (p < .001) lower than that of patients who responded. The average of non-responders was very close to that of all patients in the week prior to death. Those not responding were predominantly in or approaching the deterioration characteristic of the advanced terminal phase.

While not as dramatic, similar analyses of frequent pain, nausea, and dyspnea also revealed an overrepresentation of non-responders: 55% of non-responders versus 47% of responders were said to have frequent pain at the third interview, 47% versus 40% for nausea, and 58% versus 49% for dyspnea. Similarly, observations of level of awareness and selected other symptoms suggested that patients not responding to psychosocial questions did so because they were too sick.

Predictors of Mood State Response and Level

A series of multivariate analyses were performed to examine factors related to whether patients responded to the mood questions and, if so, the scale score obtained. The first

Table 2

Average Karnofsky Performance Status of Living Patients

Who Did and Didn't Complete the Self-Esteem Battery at Each Interview

	Patient Completed Self-Esteem Battery	
	Yes	No
First Interview	39.3	29.8
Second Interview	38.9	27.9
Third Interview	38.6	26.8
Fourth Interview	37.8	27.6
Fifth Interview	38.1	27.7
Sixth Interview	38.6	27.8
Seventh Interview	37.1	27.4

analysis used multivariate logistic regression to ascertain which of a series of factors exerted the greatest influence on whether a patient responded to the mood state questions. The second used standard multiple linear regression to achieve the same end. Identical sets of predictor variables were included in the two equations in order to compare factors associated with item response and those associated with the level of depression among those responding. The dependent variable (the abbreviated POMS depression scale) in both cases pertained to the first interview in order to maximize the sample size for the regression analysis. Similar findings were observed for subsequent interviews.

The results of the two equations are presented in Table 3. The principal predictors of being able to respond to the interview items related to patients' physical health. The lower a patient's Karnofsky Scale, the less likely it is that he/she would have responded to the mood state items. Not surprisingly, patients closer to death were less likely to respond. Interestingly, older patients were *more* likely to respond than were younger patients, controlling for performance status. Patients' outlook as judged by their PCP was strongly related to being able to respond to mood state items, a relationship primarily evident for patients rated as non-communicative.

In contrast, physical dimensions did *not* appear to be related to level of mood. The principal predictor was observer (PCP) judged outlook. Patients judged to have a positive outlook had significantly less disturbed mood scores than those patients judged to have a poor outlook. Neither patients' age, sex, nor performance status was related to mood state.

SUMMARY AND DISCUSSION

The current paper has explored a series of measurement and conceptual issues relevant to assessing whether hospice programs attain their stated goals. Analyses of the National Hospice Study (NHS) data base revealed that considerable care is required in interpreting the results of psychosocial measures taken of hospice patients, due to both the difficulties in obtaining responses and the lack of variation among responders. Comparisons of those who did and did not re-

Table 3

Multiple Logistic and Linear Regression Models

Testing the Effect of Demographic, Functional, and Symptom Variables

On the Probability of Responding to a Depression Scale

And the Level of Depression Among Respondents

	Logistic Regression Coefficients 1 = Responded 0 = Non-Response	Linear Regression Coefficients low = depressed
Pain (1=yes; 0=no)	.133	−.07
Dyspnea (1=yes; 0=no)	−.009	−.08*
Lives With PCP (1=yes; 2=no)	.060	.05
Karnofsky (low=poor)	−.053***	.04
PCP Judged Outlook (2=positive; 1=low; 0=unconscious)	.615***	.21***
Sex (1=male; 2=female)	−.102	.00
Length of Hospice Stay	−.007***	.03
Age	.017**	.03

*p < .05
**p < .01
***p < .001

spond to the mood state questions revealed that non-responders were consistently sicker and more likely to be experiencing symptoms. The high attrition rate associated with hospice patients' relatively short length of stay means that the group of patients for whom psychosocial measures can be taken will be a biased sample of the population of all hospice admissions.

How well do the NHS analyses help us address the issues raised at the outset of this paper regarding the measurement of psychosocial status among hospice patients? The paragraphs below will review the results in light of 5 issues discussed and will suggest a hierarchy of relevant quality of life constructs for the terminal cancer patient in hospice.

Using standardized scales to measure psychosocial status can yield very misleading results when applied to the hospice context. Use of even a subset of the POMS depression component revealed little variation and no change as death approached. Either these patients were calmly accepting their death, or the concept of depression as presently measured is not applicable to a physically ill, terminal population. Indeed, it has been reported that depression is difficult to diagnose in the face of serious medical illness (Goldberg, 1980). Insofar as the dominant reality for the hospice population is their imminent death and their experience of symptoms, patterns of response to and correlation with more psychiatrically oriented measures are likely to be ill fitting.

The multiplicity of psychosocial domains presents substantial complications for those interested in using extensive standardized scales to measure multi-dimensional mood and quality of life constructs. Performance status, pain and symptoms, cognitive functioning, and mood state are all relatively independent dimensions of psychosocial status. Nonetheless, in a terminal population, the various measures are observed to covary over time, suggesting that patients' status in some dimensions may be dependent upon those in another dimension. As we have seen, the most salient dynamic associated with the measurement of terminally ill patients in the present data was declining performance status and cognitive functioning.

The effect of non-response on the assessment of psychosocial status has rarely been discussed in the literature dealing with advanced cancer patients. Generally speaking, such research involved only cross-sectional interview contacts, excluding those incapable of signing consent. The NHS found the effect of missing data on the determination of psychosocial status to be present and substantial from the outset. Sicker patients were therefore unrepresented in the average mood state scores.

The PCP as data source has been proposed as valid with respect to the functioning and overall quality of life of hospice patients. Nonetheless, we made no effort to ascertain from the PCP the patient's mood state. Rather, we asked the PCP to use a variety of rating scale techniques to comment upon the status of the patient in areas ranging from pain and symptoms to cognitive capacity and outlook. These parameters were found to be moderately correlated at any point in time, but more importantly, they covaried as the patient deteriorated and approached death (Morris, Mor, et al., 1986). This suggests that the PCP can be used as a valid source of information about the patient's condition. We observed significant although moderate correlations between the patient's and the PCP's perspectives when both were available in terms of pain and outlook.

Matching measure to population is particularly difficult in the case of hospice patients and the hospice model of care. Only relatively long-stay hospice patients are likely to be able to respond to repeated evaluations of their psychosocial status. As patients deteriorate, and perhaps begin experiencing fear and a sense of isolation, they also tend to have increased somatic symptoms that are likely to overshadow the relevance of the psychosocial concerns. A large proportion of hospice patients enter the system of care already quite ill and in substantial need of symptom control interventions. The alertness and energy required to complete a detailed questionnaire or sit through what might otherwise be a pleasant interview conversation appear to be beyond the capacity of the majority of patients as death approaches. The fact that non-responders were substantially sicker than were responders at any point in time again suggests that self-reported measures of psychosocial status would not reflect the population of patients served.

A *Hierarchy of Quality of Life Measures for Hospice Research and Intervention*

The review of findings presented above suggests a model for making decisions about what aspects of hospice patients' quality of life should be measured to assess program effectiveness. Since the most prominent feature of deterioration is decline in performance status and cognitive functioning, measures of these conditions should be paramount. They should be taken preferably from the family or other non-staff caretaker in a position to observe the patient throughout most of the day. These data provide an important backdrop for understanding the process of patient deterioration. They can be used as a benchmark of optimal sustained independent functioning, presumably a goal of all hospice programs.

It is the human technology of preventive pain and symptom control that has made hospice so unique and helped it to find an important niche in the health care sector. Attention to this goal and its measurement is crucial. Data from the NHS suggest that pain and symptom control is one area in which the hospice model of intervention can really have an impact upon the lives of patients (Greer et al., in press). Continued emphasis upon performance status, pain control, and cognitive functioning are applicable to all hospice patients regardless of their length of stay. All these measures can be obtained from the PCP.

Measuring psychosocial status, as we have seen, presents considerable difficulties. Response rates are lowest at a point when the largest proportion of patients are served by hospice— close to the point of death. While psychosocial status is clearly an important issue, mood state cannot be validly evaluated in the face of distressing symptoms nor in the face of cognitive impairment due to either metastases, fatigue, or medication effects. We have seen that assessments of the patients' quality of life and particularly outlook are related to performance status as well as mood state. While the relationships are only moderate, it does suggest that a reliable approach to measuring psychosocial state may be possible by using the PCP as an informant.

Other self-report measures that specifically address the fears and anxieties said to affect the terminal patient need to be developed specifically for this population. Existing tests cannot be applied. Application of new tests, however, will always be hampered by the fact that only a portion of the hospice population will be able to respond. To the extent that they are undertaken, psychosocially oriented interventions will, however, apply to the majority of the population. Consequently, more widely applicable measures of outcome are needed.

The resulting hierarchy places both measurement and intervention emphasis upon performance status, general quality of life, and symptom control. When patients' optimal status in these areas has been facilitated, interventions directed exclusively toward improving other psychosocial states have a chance of being effective. As such, stabilization or predictability of functioning and symptom control are prerequisite to adequate assessment and intervention into patients' mood state and psychological functioning.

REFERENCES

Campbell, D.T. (1975). Reforms as experiments. In E. Struening, & M. Guttentag (Eds.), *Handbook of Evaluation Research*. Beverly Hills, CA: Sage Publications.

Cassileth, B.R., Lusk, E.J., Strouse, T.B., Miller, D.S., Brown, L.L., & Cross, P.A. (1985). A psychological analysis of cancer patients and their next-of-kin. *Cancer, 55*, 72–76.

Craig, W.G., & Abeloff, M.D. (1974). Psychiatric symptomatology among hospitalized cancer patients. *American Journal of Psychiatry, 131*, 1323–1327.

Derogatis, L.R., Morrow, G.R., Fetting, J., Penman, D., Piasetsky, S., Schmale, A.M., Henrichs, M., & Carnicke, C.L.M. (1983). The prevalence of psychiatric disorders among cancer patients. *Journal of the American Medical Association, 249*, 751–757.

Goldberg, R.J. (1980). *Strategies in Psychiatry for the Primary Physician*. Darien, CT: Patient Care Publications.

Goldberg, R.J., Wool, M.S., Glicksman, A., & Tull, R. (1984). Relationship of the social environment and patients' physical status to depression in lung cancer patients and their spouses. *Journal of Psychosocial Oncology, 2* (3/4), 73–80.

Gotay, C.C. (1984). The experience of cancer during early and advanced stages: The views of patients and their mates. *Social Science Medicine, 18* (7), 605–613.

Greer, D.S., Mor, V., & Kastenbaum, R., (Eds.) (in press). *The Hospice Experiment: Is it Working?* Baltimore, MD: Johns Hopkins University Press.

Greer, D.S., Mor, V., Morris, J.N., Sherwood, S., Kidder, D., & Birnbaum, H. (1986). An alternative in terminal care: Results of the National Hospice Study. *Journal of Chronic Diseases*.

Greer, D.S., Mor, V., Sherwood, S., Morris, J.N., & Birnbaum, H. (1983). National Hospice Study analysis plan. *Journal of Chronic Diseases, 36* (11), 737–780.

Karnofsky, D.A., Abelman, W.H., Craver, L.F., & Burchenal, J.H. (1948). The use of nitrogen mustards in the palliative treatment of carcinoma. *Cancer, 1*, 634–656.

Lawton, M.P., Whelihan, W.M., & Belsky, J.K. (1980). Personality tests and their uses with older adults. In J.E. Birren, & R.B. Sloane (Eds.), *Handbook of Mental Health and Aging*. Englewood Cliffs, NJ: Prentice-Hall.

Linn, M.W., Linn, B.S., & Harris, R. (1980). *Humanistic Oncology: The Potential in the Omega Experience*. Miami, FL: VA Medical Center.

McNair, D.M., Lorr, M., & Droppleman, L.F. (1981). *EITS Manual for the Profile of Mood States*. San Diego, CA: Educational and Industrial Testing Services.

Melzack, R. (1975). The McGill pain questionnaire: Major properties and scoring methods. *Pain, 1*, 277–299.

Mor, V. (in press). *Hospice Literature: A Critical Review of the Process, Outcome, and Costs of Care*. New York, NY: Springer Publications.

Mor, V., Laliberte, L., Morris, J.N., & Wiemann, M. (1984). The Karnofsky performance status scale: An examination of its reliability and validity in a research setting. *Cancer, 53* (9), 2002–2007.

Morris, J.N., Mor, V., Goldberg, R.J., Sherwood, S., Greer, D.S., & Hiris, J. (1986). The effect of treatment setting and patient characteristics on pain in terminal cancer patients: A report from the National Hospice Study. *Journal of Chronic Diseases*.

Morris, J.N., Suizza, S., Sherwood, S., Wright, S.M., & Greer, D.S. (1986). Last

Days: A study of the quality of life of terminally ill cancer patients. *Journal of Chronic Diseases.*

National Hospice Organization (1979). *Standards of a Hospice Program of Care.* McLean, VA: NHO.

Nunnally, J.C. (1967). *Psychometric Theory.* New York, NY: McGraw-Hill.

Oleson, T.D., & Bresler, D.E. (1979). California pain assessment profile. In T.D. Oleson, & R. Turbo (Eds.), *Free Yourself From Pain.* New York, NY: Simon and Schuster.

Peck, A. (1972). Emotional reactions to having cancer. *American Journal of Roentgenology, 114,* 591–599.

Plumb, M.M., & Holland, J. (1977). Comparative studies of psychological function in patients with advanced cancer-I. Self-reported depressive symptoms. *Psychosomatic Medicine, 39* (4), 264–276.

Rosenberg, M. (1973). In J.P. Robinson, & P.R. Shaver (Eds.), *Measures of Social Psychological Attitudes.* Ann Arbor, MI: Institute of Social Research, University of Michigan.

Sechrest, L. (1985). Observer studies: Data collection by remote control. In L. Burstein, H.E. Freeman, & P.H. Rossi (Eds.), *Collecting Evaluation Data.* Beverly Hills, CA: Sage Publications, Inc.

Spitzer, W.O., Dobson, A.J., Hall, J., Chesterman, E., Levi, J., Shepherd, R., & Catchlove, B. (1981). Measuring the quality of life of cancer patients: A concise QL index for use by physicians. *Journal of Chronic Diseases, 34,* 585–597.

Biopsychosocial Assessment of Cancer Patients: Methods and Suggestions

Patricia L. Dobkin
Gary R. Morrow

ABSTRACT. Assessment of biopsychosocial factors in cancer patients is presented with an emphasis on methodological issues. Typical cancer patient problems are identified (e.g., depression, pain, nausea and vomiting) and various means of evaluating these are discussed. Types and criteria for assessment are briefly outlined so as to enable the reader to critique methods currently in use. Pertinent issues in psychosocial oncology assessment such as patient definition, assessment timing, and relevancy of assessment are addressed, as are considerations concerning the sensitive use of clinical judgment when working with this population. It was concluded that instruments and procedures employed should be relatively brief and that they need to be chosen judicially. Finally, the clinician's understanding, sensitivity and empathy are viewed as paramount to accurate, comprehensive biopsychosocial assessment of cancer patients.

Historically cancer research has been focused on biomedical issues such as etiology and cancer treatment while less immediate problems, such as psychosocial consequences of disease, have received relatively little attention. In the 1950's, investigations with cancer patients which did include psychological variables attempted (without success) to demonstrate a causal link between certain personality factors and the devel-

Gary R. Morrow, PhD, is an associate professor of Oncology and Psychiatry. Patricia L. Dobkin, MS, is an intern in Psychosocial Oncology and Clinical Psychology. Supported in part by grants CA 11198, CA 26832 and Research Cancer Developments Award CA 01038 from the National Cancer Institute, DHHS and by grant PDT 217 from the American Cancer Society. Mailing address: University of Rochester Cancer Center, 601 Elmwood Avenue, Box 704, Rochester, New York 14642.

opment of specific cancers. Later work has addressed treatment related questions such as whether or not to inform patients of their diagnosis. More recently, research has been directed at such areas as helping patients adapt to treatment effects (e.g., mastectomy), and to increase knowledge of informed consent (Morrow, Gootnick, & Schmale, 1978).

In a reasonably short period, psychosocial oncology has developed into a broad field which encompasses aspects of cancer disease, its treatment, and the impact it has on the patient.

Typical problems experienced by cancer patients have been identified. For instance, upon learning of diagnosis or poor prognosis, some cancer patients become depressed. Many patients are extremely anxious about their symptomatology and treatments; others are angry about their fate. In addition to emotional distress, cancer patients may exhibit behavioral problems. For example, conditioned responses such as anticipatory nausea and vomiting in chemotherapy patients (i.e., becoming ill prior to treatment) or avoidance of medical procedures due to fear are recognized by health professionals as significant problems (Morrow, Arseneau, Asbury, Bennett, & Boros, 1982). In addition, some patients develop "psychosomatic symptoms" which potentially complicate treatment implementation (Redd, Rosenberger, & Hendler, 1983).

The cancer experience fundamentally disrupts a patient and his/her family's lifestyle. Future plans are arrested, roles are reversed, financial reserves are spent, and many things suddenly seem to be so unpredictable. These abrupt changes may have a profound impact on all individuals involved with the patient along with the patient.

A patient's experience of the cancer process may influence response to treatment and subsequent quality of life. We (Morrow, 1980) and others such as Holland (1984) have pointed out that few psychosocial assessment instruments are appropriate for assessment of cancer patients. Most available measures have been designed for physically healthy, psychiatrically impaired patients. These instruments thus may require modification in order to be used with cancer patients.

Here we focus on a pragmatic view of the psychosocial assessment of cancer patients. Following a brief outline of types and criteria for assessment, available instruments and procedures are discussed in a representative, rather than exhaustive, review and critique. Important assessment issues are discussed with an emphasis on the practical considerations necessary when working with an advanced cancer population.

ASSESSMENT OF BIOPSYCHOSOCIAL FACTORS

Types of Assessment

Assessment encompasses a wide domain with various "schools of thought" (e.g., psychodynamic, humanistic) that emphasize different techniques. There are four principle means of assessment: self-report, direct observation, physiological recording, and indirect measure. These methods can be employed singularly or in combination. Each has both advantages and disadvantages.

Self-report involves having an individual disclose his/her perception of that which is being measured. This may be accomplished through an *interview,* completion of a *survey,* or by having the person self-rate or *self-monitor* the construct in question. Self-report methods are perhaps the most frequently used assessment tools in general practice since they are relatively easy to administer, cost-effective, and may be used with a large sample. A prominent problem with this approach is that it is potentially unreliable. Many factors such as reactivity (e.g., experimenter effect, social desirability), ignorance, or even a misunderstanding of instructions may have an effect on findings. Self-report is thus an important, but not always sufficient, means of information gathering. Self-report data are strengthened by corroboration from other sources.

Direct observation involves having the investigator (or a trained collaborator) record specific response occurrence. Data collection may be performed in either a natural environment (e.g., at home) or in contrived (analogue) situations. For instance, one may have a spouse record the number of times his/her wife/husband dresses a wound postoperatively. Direct observation may be subject to fewer biases than self-report but it is not without disadvantages. Reactivity and observer bias may distort findings. Observers must be carefully trained and reliability checks need to be made in order to ensure accuracy (see Kent & Foster, 1977, for a thorough discussion of this assessment method).

Many investigators consider *psychophysiological* measures to be the most sophisticated means of psychological assessment. An advantage of this approach is that data yield is presumably maximized while data biases are minimized; a potential problem is that these data may easily be misinterpreted. An investigator needs expertise in psychophysiology to accurately interpret findings. Too often a single measure is taken out of the context of a dynamic physiological system. A second problem with psychophysiological assessment involves its cost. Few clinicians have at their disposal the expensive equipment required for accurate data collection of this type.

A final type of assessment involves *indirect* measures. Behavioral changes may be inferred from presumably related measures. For example, urine analysis may indicate drug usage or weight loss may suggest adherence to a diet.

Behavioral assessment is a relatively new approach to analyzing maladaptive patterns of behavior. A brief account will be outlined. More complete reviews have been given by Ciminero, Calhoun, and Adams (1977), and the following discussion is based on Kanfer and Saslow's (1969) S-O-R-C-K model. A functional analysis is carried out in order to determine antecedent stimuli (S) which affect an organism (O) who responds in a certain manner (R) with both consequences of that response (C) and contingencies which maintain it (K). As an example, a cancer patient (O) may enter a chemotherapy clinic and see an oncology nurse (S) and suddenly experience nausea (R). Consequently, the patient comes to dread his/her treatments (C). The contingencies (K) in this example are related to a learning process which underlies the development of the response.

Behavioral assessment may be accomplished through the combination of the four general approaches previously discussed, namely: self-report, direct and indirect behavioral observations, and physiological recordings. The advantage of this approach is that it leads directly to treatment selection and evaluation of treatment progress. Its major drawback is a product of the inevitability that the more an assessment approach is tailored to the individual, the more difficult it is to standardize across individuals.

Criteria for Assessment

Assessment is rendered meaningless if it does not accurately reflect that which is purportedly being measured. Psychometric issues in assessment become relevant when observations are transformed into numerical scores or when inferences are drawn from observed behavior (see Goldfried & Lineham, 1977). A brief review of essential criteria for assessment will be presented here as a basis for the subsequent section concerning procedures and instruments used to assess cancer patients' experiences.

The most important criteria for assessment are:

a. Validity
b. Reliability
c. Standardization
d. Norms
e. Clinical utility
f. Coverage

Validity comes in many forms and is an essential aspect of accurate measurement; it concerns the essence of what is being measured. There are basically three forms of validity: content, construct, and criterion-related (also termed concurrent) validity. The degree to which an instrument or approach is accepted as valid is a reflection on the degree to which it seems to measure that which it purports to measure. In general, a programmatic line of research is required to determine whether or not an instrument is valid.

Reliability is another important yardstick in assessment. It refers to the consistency of measurement. Derogatis and Spencer (1984) describe reliability as the converse of measurement error. Standardization of the measurement process can increase reliability. If the administration of a test differs across patients, one can hardly draw convincing conclusions from the results found. In self-report data collection, standardization can be accomplished through the use of structured interviews, forced-choice questionnaires, or by preprinted self-monitoring forms. In direct observation data collection, observers can be trained to complete preprinted rating forms. In psychophysiological measurement, procedures used and instrumentation can be set up in a specific manner to insure that each patient response is measured consistently.

Norms are relevant in assessment because they provide a point of reference. Behavior is "abnormal" only with regard to a group standard. In psychosocial oncology it can be difficult to discern what is normal. Should one compare a depressed cancer patient to a healthy individual or a patient with a different illness? Derogatis and Spencer (1984) note that specific problems arise when seeking a normative sample for a cancer population because numerous factors (e.g., diagnosis, stage and duration of illness, prognosis) can influence characteristics relevant to assessment. Age and gender in particular may influence psychological responses. There is no simple solution to the norm question. Generally, normative data which best suits the hypothesis being tested is the appropriate comparison.

Clinical utility is an assessment issue which may appear to be obvious but is quite often overlooked. The purposes of assessment are (a) to determine the nature of a problem, (b) to select an intervention for that problem, and (c) to evaluate the effectiveness of the intervention employed. In an advanced cancer population there may be no rationale for assessing certain variables if all treatment options in the given problem area have been exhausted. Discretion and clinical judgment are essential in determining whether or not assessment is appropriate.

Coverage in assessment refers to inclusiveness. It maintains an inverse relationship with specificity. If a test provides information concerning a vast array of responses it may be difficult to draw specific conclusions from the findings. On the other hand, if a test is too circumscribed it may be impossible to generalize the findings. Ideally, one should gather enough data so that something is learned but restrict measurement sufficiently so that findings can be interpreted parsimoniously.

PSYCHOSOCIAL ASSESSMENT OF CANCER PATIENTS

Research in psychosocial oncology has shown that assessment tools need to be designed specifically for this unique population. Currently, psychological tests and questionnaires are being developed which measure general areas of cancer patients' lives such as "quality of life" or more specific aspects of the disease process such as physical and psychological side effects of cancer treatment. In the following section a sampling of assessment tools currently being used with cancer patients will be presented. These are summarized in Table 1.

Quality of Life

The construct "quality of life" is as difficult to define as it is to measure. Schipper et al. (1984) point out a lack of consensus on whether or not this construct is a distinct entity. Most investigators view quality of life as a composite of intrapersonal, interpersonal, occupational, and physical characteristics (e.g., see Padilla, Presant, Grant, et al., 1983).

Wellisch (1984) has suggested that at least three methodological issues need to be considered in the study of quality of life of a medical population: (a) when to make the assessment (i.e., disease stage), (b) which assessment techniques need to be used, and (c) who makes the assessment (e.g., doctor, nurse, social worker). After reviewing advantages and disadvantages of various methodological approaches in quality of life research, Wellisch advocates combining a structured interview with analogue scales and behavioral measures. As an example, he cites Sugarbaker and coworkers' (1981) study which employed (a) a semistructured interview in the form of the Psychosocial Adjustment to Illness Scale (Derogatis, 1975); (b) two measures of daily activities and functioning (Katz Activity of Daily Living Scale: Katz & Akpom, 1966; Barthel Index: Mahoney & Barthel, 1965); (c) data concerning the functional outcomes of cancer treatment (Sickness Impact Profile: Bergner, Bobbitt, Polland, Martin, & Gilson, 1976); (d) economic change indicators; and (e) clinical scales designed specifically for cancer patients relating treatment consequences to quality of life. The main problem with this comprehensive approach involves its cost; much time and energy on the part of both patient and investigator is required to complete the evaluation.

Padilla and her colleagues (1983) developed an instrument designed to measure the quality of life in cancer patients. The Quality of Life Index (QLI) is comprised of 14 linear ana-

Table 1

Examples of Instruments Used to Assess Psychosocial Problems in Oncology Patients

Instrument	Where Reported	Variable(s) Assessed
Linear Analogue Self-Assessment	Coates et al. (1983)	Quality of life
Functional Living Index	Schipper et al. (1984)	Quality of life
Quality of Life Index*	Padilla et al. (1983)	Quality of life
Cancer Inventory of Problem Situations *	Heinrich et al. (1984)	27 categories of problems
Psychosocial Problem Categories for Homebound Cancer Patients*	Wellisch et al. (1983)	5 main problem categories
Symptoms Checklist-90	Derogatis (1977) Farber et al. (1984)	Social adjustment
Psychosocial Adjustment to Illness	Derogatis (1977) Morrow et al. (1978)	Psychosocial adjustment
Rating of Psychosocial Function*	Morrow et al. (1981)	Coping style
Coping Adequate Rating	Morrow et al. (1981)	Coping style
Global Adjustment to Illness Scale	Morrow et al. (1981)	Adjustment to illness
Morrow Assessment of Nausea and Emesis*	Morrow (1982; 1984)	Nausea and vomiting
Wisconsin Brief Pain Questionnaire*	Daut et al. (1983)	Pain
McGill Pain Quesionnaire	Graham et al. (1980)	Pain

*Indicates that the instrument was developed specifically for cancer patients.

logue scales which assess general physical condition, normal activities, and personal attitudes towards life. Padilla et al. (1983) investigated the reliability, internal consistency, construct validity, discriminant and concurrent validity of the QLI. They found that test-retest reliability varied as a function of patient status and treatment modality (outpatient versus impatient, chemotherapy versus radiation therapy). Reportedly, reliability was highest for chemotherapy outpatients and lowest for a healthy control group. One cannot, however, determine if the QLI is reliable based on these findings because the timing of test administration differed across groups. Item analysis of the QLI resulted in an alpha reliability of .88 (p < .01), indicating good internal consistency.

Despite its simplicity and ease of administration, it appears that the QLI requires further development before it can be accepted as a useful assessment tool. Its reliability has yet to be demonstrated as does its concurrent validity. In addition, the QLI does not account for non-cancer related aspects of patients' lives which may interact with, and thereby confound, quality of life measurement.

Schipper, McMurray, and Levitt (1984) measure the quality of life in cancer patients using the Functional Living Index (FLIC). The FLIC is a self-administered 22 item questionnaire which is disease specific and functionally oriented. It can be used to evaluate trends both within and between patients. Four principal functional areas are measured: (a) vocation, (b) affect, (c) social interaction, and (d) somatic sensation. The questionnaire was developed over a series of trials in two Canadian cities with 837 cancer patients. Methods used to validate the FLIC included factor analysis, concurrent validity checks, and stratification of six groups representing broad categories of disease status.

Schipper et al. (1984) presented data which supports the view that the FLIC is a valid tool for the assessment of the quality of life in cancer patients. The authors caution that the FLIC is not "the ultimate measure" but that it can be used to provide adjunctive information in the interpretation of comparative clinical trials.

Psychosocial Adjustment

Much like quality of life, "psychosocial adjustment" is a complex and difficult construct to measure. The term psychosocial denotes an interaction between intrapersonal and interpersonal events. Adjustment concerns responding to the environment in an adaptive manner. Psychosocial adjustment in oncology refers to how the impact of having and being treated for cancer is handled by the individual. Patients often report that the cancer experience "changes their whole lives." What does this statement mean and how can such an impact be measured?

In a study involving 37 Hodgkin's disease patients and their parents, Morrow, Chiarello, and Derogatis (1978) investigated the psychometric properties of the Psychosocial Adjustment to Illness Scale (PAIS). The PAIS consists of 45 questions which are presented to the patient in a semi-structured interview format. The questions can be divided into seven relatively independent domains of functioning: (a) health care orientation, (b) vocational environment, (c) domestic environment, (d) sexual relationships, (e) extended family relationships, (f) social environment, and (g) psychological distress. Significant correlations between subscales of the PAIS and such psychological tests as the State Trait Anxiety Inventory, Beck Depression Inventory, and Symptom Checklist-90 suggest that the PAIS is a valid tool. Interrater reliability was sufficiently high ($r = 0.83$) to support the contention that despite its interview format, the PAIS is an acceptable means of assessing psychosocial adjustment. The authors concluded that although replication is required, the PAIS can be administered with an acceptable level of confidence in its reliability and validity.

In a more recent study, Morrow, Feldstein, Adler, et al. (1981) evaluated five brief instruments designed to measure psychosocial adjustment to medical illness (Rating of Psychosocial Function (RPF): Holland, 1976; Global Adjustment to Illness Scale (GAIS): Derogatis, 1976; Coping Strategies Inventory (CSI): Weissman, 1975; Coping Adequacy Rating (CAR): Balinsky & Berger, 1975; Rochester Psychosocial State Evaluation Form (RPSEF): Berg, 1976). These five instruments were administered to cancer patients by 105 health professionals (nurses, oncologists, social workers, psychologists) in five separate cancer centers. The instruments were selected based on three criteria: (a) brevity of test administration time, (b) global rating of patient status required (less than five minutes), and (c) conceptual relevance (i.e., construct validity).

Morrow and his coworkers (1981) videotaped the interviews and evaluated the instruments in terms of the time and effort required to complete them, the effects of rater experience on interrater reliability, and the effect of the raters' professional training on reliability. The RPF, CAR, and GAIS were found to be highly interrelated and most favorably supported by the data. This finding suggests a degree of overlap supporting convergent validity. Discriminant validity was supported by a reasonable divergence of indices across psychological domains. Agreement on ratings was not influenced by the length of the interview but appeared to be affected by the structure of the interview and profession of the raters (nurse, social worker, etc.). All three instruments showed a relationship with clinical impressions, indicating concurrent validity. The GAIS was chosen as most adequate reflection of a clinical impression by the majority of raters. The authors concluded that, with adequate training, any of the three instruments could be used to assess psychosocial adjustment in cancer patients.

Affect

Cancer patients are a largely nonpsychiatric, heterogeneous group of individuals experiencing a health crisis. How patients respond to this extremely stressful situation may vary as a function of many factors. The stage of the disease process (diagnosis, treatment, remission, etc.), and individual's particular coping style, available social supports, and physical well-being potentially contribute to how a patient reacts. Typically cancer patients experience a high level of anxiety during the initial stages of treatment and during difficult treatment procedures. Depression is a common response with disease recurrence. Generally, health professionals determine patients' affective responses based on "clinical judgement"; this, however, is only a rough index of what patients are experiencing.

Endicott (1984) proposed the use of scaled measures for the assessment of depression in cancer patients. She utilizes revisions of the standard (DSM III) criteria for classification of Major Depression in a medical population. As an example, "fearfulness or depressed appearance in face or body posture" are substituted for more easily misleading vegetative signs such as appetite and weight changes. In this way, the fact that anorexia or weight gain often occur as a result of cancer and its treatment is taken into account.

Gottschalk (1984) specifies three variables which are important to consider when measuring affect in cancer patients. The first factor, direct effects of the disease, (e.g., an endocrine-producing tumor) may result in behavior which mimics depressive symptoms. The second factor, indirect effects, (e.g., aversive side effects of cancer treatment) may also influence a patient's affective state. For instance, it may be difficult to discern if fatigue is the result of cancer treatment or of psychological factors. Or, one could easily suppose that the patient is "just a nervous person" when, in fact, she or he is fearful of a specific medical procedure. The fact that cancer patients may be given psychoactive pharmacologic agents for non-psychiatric problems (e.g., compazine for nausea/emesis) is also relevant here. The side effects of these drugs may produce affect-related symptoms. Finally, the natural course of cancer may have a profound effect on a patient's response. Not surprisingly, depression may "spontaneously remit" when treatment is terminated with good prognosis or worsen when it is determined that cure is not possible.

Cognitions

Problems of a cognitive nature resulting from cancer and its treatment have received relatively little attention. Recently, Folstein, Fetting, Lobo, et al. (1984) reported that almost one-third of the oncology inpatients they measured on the Mini-Mental Status Examination were cognitively impaired. Since cognitive impairment may be the result of severe metabolic imbalances (Wolff & Curran, 1955) the biomedical etiology of dysfunction requires clarification.

Much like affect, cognitive functioning should be assessed in the general context of a patient's overall medical status and psychological state. An elderly person in acute pain may perform poorly on a test due to fatigue rather than incapacity. A depressed parent preoccupied with child care problems may respond in a distracted manner. These potentially confounding factors need to be acknowledged and taken into account to accurately assess cognitive abilities. Once impairment is indicated, it is important to define the associated syndrome.

Folstein et al. (1984) administered a brief bedside battery of tests to assess cognitive functioning in cancer patients. One test in the battery, the linear analogue scale of consciousness, is simple to use with acceptable interrater reliability (r's = .81

to .97). The scale rates consciousness on a 0 to 10 cm scale (from very drowsy (0) to normally alert (10)). A second test, a hand held Tachistoscope, is employed in order to determine the patient's ability to perceive stimuli. Delirious patients are unable to perform this task within normal time limits (1/60th second). Perception time will thus identify most clinically delirious cancer patients. The third test in the battery is the Mini-Mental State Examination (MMSE: Folstein, Folstein, & McHugh, 1975) which assesses (a) orientation, (b) registration, (c) attention and calculation, (d) recall, and (e) language. The MMSE is derived from the National Institute of Mental Health Diagnostic Interview. The original diagnostic interview has been administered to a normative sample of approximately 15,000 individuals in five geographic locations.

This test battery is claimed to enable the examiner to assess delirium according to DSM III criteria (Folstein et al., 1984). However, numerous factors such as fatigue, medical status, age, drug usage (to name just a few) may distort test scores. Another weakness of this approach is that the test battery measures essentially *gross* cognitive functioning, which may be more parsimoniously assessed by clinical interview (Silberfarb, 1984).

Silberfarb, Philibert, and Levine (1980) advocate using a different set of procedures to assess cognitive deficits in cancer patients. Interestingly, these authors measure affective responses in conjunction with cognitions in order to account for potential interactions between these variables. Patient examination lasts approximately 30–60 minutes and involves (a) The Cognitive Capacity Screening Test, a standardized mental status exam; (b) The Trail Making B Test; and (c) The Digit Symbol Test, a subtest of the Wechsler Adult Intelligence Scale. The latter two tests have been shown to be quite sensitive in detecting brain damage (Reitan, 1955; 1958). In a study of 50 medical oncology patients, Silberfarb et al. found that impaired cognition was quite common, independent of affective responses. Notably, patients treated with chemotherapy were more likely than any other group to be cognitively impaired.

Silverfarb's battery (1980) seems more practical and comprehensive than Folstein and his coworkers' (1984) assessment of delirium—only one of several types of cognitive deficit evident in cancer patients. Examiners investigating cognitive functioning should be well-versed in neuropsychology and brain-behavior relationships in order to accurately interpret their findings.

Pain

Pain is a distressing and debilitating problem for many cancer patients. Research shows that one-third of adult cancer patients experience pain in the non-terminal stage and as many as two-thirds of dying patients are in some degree of pain during the terminal stage of illness (Foley, 1984). Foley (1984) classifies cancer pain as follows: (1) acute, cancer-related; (2) chronic, cancer-related; (3) preexisting chronic in addition to cancer-related pain; and (4) pain in terminal patients. Acute cancer pain may be associated with the diagnosis of cancer (i.e., a presenting symptom) and/or with cancer treatment. Chronic pain may be associated with cancer treatment and disease progression. Foley emphasizes that the clinician assessing cancer pain needs to have a solid background in oncology in order to be able to recognize clinical syndromes that signal metastasis. She advocates that clinical assessment of pain involve adherence to nine principles:

1. Believing in the patient's pain complaint
2. Taking a careful history of the pain complaint
3. Assessing the psychosocial status of the patient
4. Performing a careful medical and neurological examination
5. Ordering and personally reviewing the appropriate diagnostic procedures
6. Evaluating the extent of the patient's disease
7. Treating the pain to facilitate the diagnostic study
8. Considering alternative methods to pain control during the initial evaluation
9. Reassessing the pain complaint during the prescribed therapy (Foley, 1984, p. 22).

This approach relies heavily, of necessity, on clinical judgement. Usually examiners ask patients to rate pain intensity in terms of categories (e.g., "none", "slight", "moderate", "severe", "intolerable"), or on a numerical rating scale (e.g., 0 to 10, where 0 indicates no pain and 10 indicates excruciating pain). As an alternative, Wallenstein (1984) suggests using the Visual Analogue Scale (VAS) to measure pain. The VAS consists of a 10 cm line drawn on a page with the words "least possible pain" and "worst possible pain" on the two ends of the continuum. The patient is requested to place a mark on the line in order to indicate his/her pain level. Wallenstein and his coworkers (Wallenstein, Rogers, Kaiko, Hendrich, & Houde, 1980) propose that the VAS is a reliable instrument which is more sensitive than rating scales (both numerical and categories) and more acceptable to patients. The shortcoming of the VAS is that it measures only one aspect of the pain experience, namely intensity. Therefore, it is recommended that the VAS be used in conjunction with other measures.

Graham, Bond, Gerkovich, and Cook (1980) have used the McGill Pain Questionnaire (MPQ: Melzack, 1975) in order to provide quantitative data concerning pain in cancer patients. The MPQ is an attractive assessment instrument for several reasons. First of all, it is easy to administer and is cost-efficient. Secondly, it categorizes pain into three dimensions (sensory, affective and evaluative). Another feature of the MPQ is that it can be used to assess the effectiveness of pain intervention. The MPQ is, however, an imperfect instrument. Since the number of categories per dimension and the number of words per category are not proportionally distributed, statistical analyses performed on MPQ data may result in inaccurate data. Another inherent problem of the MPQ concerns its language use; the adjectives included on the questionnaire may be too difficult for patients without a college education to comprehend. Finally, Melzack (1975) and Graham et al. (1980) suggest that the MPQ reflects current pain levels rather than a summary of pain over a specified period of time. While the MPQ may be clinically useful, it appears of restricted value for research purposes.

The Wisconsin Brief Pain Questionnaire (BPQ) is a newly devised, self-administered questionnaire developed by Daut, Cleeland, and Flanery (1983). The BPQ focuses on several aspects of pain: history, intensity, location, quality, cause, and interference with activities. It represents a compromise between coverage and inherent limitations imposed by a medically ill population. While it is important to recognize the complex nature of pain perception, one should not demand too much time or energy from patients who are experiencing discomfort.

In a test of the psychometric qualities of the BPQ, 1200 consecutive in- and outpatients at the Wisconsin Clinical Cancer Center were studied. In order to limit variation in type and severity of pain, patients were selected with cancer at four primary sites (breast, prostate, colon-rectal, and gynecological). Significant correlations were found for high pain ratings and the use of pain relievers. High pain ratings also correlated significantly with activity interference and mood. These results suggest that the BPQ is a valid instrument.

Reliability of the BPQ was assessed by readministering the test to two groups. One group was retested over a short period of time (M = 1.9 days). A second group was retested over an extended period of time (M = 91.4 days). Not surprisingly, the test-retest correlation were higher for the former group. This finding may reflect either poor reliability over longer periods, or actual temporal fluctuations in pain levels as measured by the BPQ. Overall, the BPQ appears to be a useful means of measuring pain. But, as the authors caution, no single instrument can adequately assess all relevant aspects of pain. The BPQ does not gather information on the emotional significance of pain nor on the situational determinants of pain behavior.

Nausea and Vomiting

A recent study reviewed over 120 studies that included assessment of nausea and emesis as a portion of their outcome measures for 1512 cancer patients (Morrow, 1984). Key issues discussed were: (a) definition of response terms, (b) self-report *versus* observer-rated assessment, (c) the usefulness of both direct and indirect assessments of nausea and emesis, (d) whether combining nausea and vomiting responses into overall measures is justified, (e) timing in assessing postchemotherapy nausea and vomiting, and (f) the need to include measures of anticipatory nausea/emesis in an assessment schema.

Morrow (1984) notes that there may be as many scales for

assessing nausea/vomiting as there are researchers studying the phenomenon. Different investigators have used different criteria in developing overall ratings. Morrow consolidates the many viewpoints with the following suggestions: (1) The assessment of nausea (including frequency, duration, severity) should be separate from the assessment of vomiting. (2) When assessing change in nausea and emesis it is important to select a consistent time frame that makes sense clinically. (3) The use of observer-rated measures is an appropriate assessment strategy for the frequency of vomiting. Its accuracy in nausea assessment, however, may be suspect. In addition, one should employ two independent raters whenever possible to allow for reliability checks. (4) Anticipatory nausea/emesis assessment needs to be included in studies involving cancer chemotherapy patients.

Morrow has developed the Morrow Assessment of Nausea and Emesis (MANE), a self-administered questionnaire that includes distinct questions concerning anticipatory nausea, anticipatory vomiting, postchemotherapy nausea, and post-chemotherapy vomiting. Specific parameters of nausea and vomiting (i.e., frequency, duration, and severity) are also measured. Content validity of the MANE was supported by the finding that patient-reported anticipatory symptoms and posttreatment side effects were statistically unrelated. A general pattern of independence among the topographic elements of nausea and vomiting supported their inclusion in the scale as distinct phenomena. Convergent validity was supported by the finding that independent measures associated with nausea and vomiting were more highly correlated with the MANE than with measures of other chemotherapy side effects. The scale was shown to be sensitive to changes in emetogenic chemotherapy drugs in that a change in drug protocol was reflected in changes in scale values. Test-retest reliability correlations for the MANE ranged from .72 to .96 for four consecutive treatments cycles. These results provide support for the view that the MANE reliably assesses patient-reported nausea and vomiting. An initial degree of confidence appears warranted concerning the MANE's validity. The future employment of the MANE should be determined by its support in independent study by other investigators.

Ahles and his coworkers (Ahles, Cohen, Little, Balducci,

Dubbert, & Keane, 1984) describe a practical, unobtrusive method for conducting a trimodal assessment of anticipatory nausea and vomiting. In a recent pilot study, nine cancer patients receiving chemotherapy were selected by the staff oncology nurse. Three presented with postchemotherapy nausea and vomiting (PCNV), three with anticipatory nausea and vomiting (ANV) and three with anticipatory nausea without vomiting (AN). The diagnosis and treatment regimens administered varied across patients. Patients' responses were measured using the following procedures: (1) MANE, (2) VAS for nausea and anxiety, and (3) experimenter-observed emesis. Heart rate was recorded using an unobtrusive monitoring device (Respironics Inc., Model EX-3 Excentry).

Ahles et al. (1984) found three separate response patterns for patients undergoing cancer chemotherapy. PCNV patients reported low levels of nausea and anxiety and showed no evidence of physiological arousal. AN patients reported elevations on measures of nausea and anxiety only. ANV patients reported increased nausea and anxiety, and showed elevated levels of physiological arousal (increased heart rate and heart rate variability). Correlational data concerning the relationship between measures on the MANE and VAS for nausea were not presented. One should, however, be cautious in interpreting heart rate data out of context. Heart rate is a function of a dynamic physiological system and it is affected by many complex interacting factors.

Sexual Dysfunction

Greenberg (1984) has written a thoughtful paper on assessment of sexual dysfunction in cancer patients. She points out that since sexual behavior is simultaneously somatic, psychological, and interpersonal, it must be measured accordingly. Information regarding the patient's premorbid sexual experience, developmental stage, expectations, and relationships are required in order to understand a patient's problem. In addition, organic variables such as the severity of illness and pharmacologic agents administered need to be included in assessment so as to allow the patient's perspective to be viewed in the context of his/her disease process. The main point to keep in mind when assessing sexual (dys)function in a cancer patient population is that a biopsychosocial approach will help the examiner to understand and treat these types of problems.

Pertinent Issues in Assessment of Cancer Patients

Certain pertinent issues arise when making a psychosocial assessment in a cancer patient population. First, the disease *stage* and *status* of the patient should be clearly identified. For instance, an inpatient differs considerably from a hospice patient in terms of environmental and psychosocial factors. The *timing* of assessment is also an important measurement consideration. Patients' responses vary as a function of disease stage. Advanced cancer patients may be physically disabled, in pain, and are likely to have experienced significant emotional distress. These factors need to be considered when interpreting assessment findings.

Psychometric issues previously discussed are also relevant here. The validity and reliability of instruments and procedures used are critical to an adequate assessment of the patient. Has an instrument been modified to suit a cancer population? Are there norms with whom to compare the results? Have interviews been standardized? Importantly, is the assessment itself *relevant*? i.e., Will it lead to a better understanding of the patient and subsequent intervention selection? These questions may appear commonsensical, but they often are left either unasked or unanswered.

Relevant Considerations in Assessment of Cancer Patients

Cancer patients, especially those in the terminal stage, are physically ill and are often distressed. Assessment should be as *brief* and as *unobtrusive* as possible so as not to add to patients' difficulties. Clinical judgment must be used concerning the appropriateness of measurement techniques. Sensitivity to the situation at hand is a prerequisite to patient contact. It is often helpful to be familiar with a patient's chart prior to assessment so as to require the least amount of patient time necessary.

Certain types of cancer result in typical problems. For example, breast and prostate cancer patients often experience sexual dysfunction during or following treatment. It is logical and appropriate to select assessment methods based on diagnosis and treatment modality. A "shot-gun" approach, often seen in the form of an extensive battery of tests, may exhaust the patient and elude parsimonious explanations of findings. It is to be avoided whenever possible.

Finally, it is important to know patients' education levels and cultural backgrounds. Not all individuals understand questions on inventories nor are they accustomed to completing forms. It is the investigator's responsibility to ensure that effective communication is accomplished.

Homebound Cancer Patients

Wellish, Landsverk, Guidera, et al. (1983) studied the types and frequency of problems in advanced cancer patients and their families in a home setting by administering The Psychosocial Problem Categories for Homebound Cancer Patients. Included in the questionnaire were 70 problems which were subdivided into 13 categories. The five most frequent reported difficulties were: (a) somatic side effects (30% of total problems, of which pain involved 13%); (b) mood disturbance (15% of total problems); (c) equipment problems (8% of total problems); (d) family relationship impairment (7% of total problems); and (e) cognitive impairment (6% of total problems). Unfortunately, the methodology used in this study render these findings tentative, at best. First of all, data were amassed through chart review. Anyone who has audited medical records is aware that missing or incorrect chart data constitutes a serious problem. Secondly, when raters disagreed about how to code data they negotiated a consensual agreement. This procedure devalues the interpretability of the interrater reliability coefficient ($r = .96$). In addition, it is impossible to determine whether these findings reflect the health care professionals' perceptions and charting habits or the true experiences of cancer patients.

Wellisch et al.'s (1983) investigation does highlight the fact that it is difficult to carry out assessment in an advanced cancer patient population. The examiner must be sensitive to questions such as, "Is it ethical to intrude on a patient's (and family members') privacy at this critical stage of illness?" Patients and/or their significant others may resent being "studied" at this time or they may simply be experiencing too much stress to endure an evaluation.

The most important factor to keep in mind during clinical assessment is its purpose: to select the intervention which is most likely to alleviate suffering. In order to accomplish this goal one should carefully consider the biological, psychological, and social factors influencing the patient at the time of measurement. Clearly, experience with cancer patients aids assessment. For instance, being cognizant of which side effects are likely to occur with the various treatment modalities or knowing where metastasis often occur in particular types of cancer (e.g., lung cancer: metastasis to the brain) can aid in the selection of procedures and assessment methods.

Adequate assessment demands extensive training and experience on the part of the examiner. Patience and empathy are part of the job; patients respond best (and thereby give the most information) when they sense a caring approach. Oncology staff members are more cooperative when they feel that their patients will *benefit* from psychosocial assessment. These are hardly minor considerations. (See McCorkle, Packard, & Landenburger, 1985 for a discussion of success in psychosocial oncology research). If one wishes to collect data which accurately reflect an ongoing experience it is crucial to become an integral part of what is happening in the clinical setting.

REFERENCES

Ahles, T. A., Cohen, R. E., Little, D., Balducci, L., Dubbert, P. M., & Keane, T. M. (1984). Toward a behavioral assessment of anticipatory symptoms associated with cancer chemotherapy. *Journal of Behavior Therapy and Experimental Psychiatry, 15,* 141–145.

Balinsky, W., Berger, R. (1975). A review of the literature in general health status indexes. *Medical Care, 13,* 283–293.

Bergner, M., Bobbit, R. A., Pollard, W. E., Martin, D. P., & Gilson, B. S. (1976). The sickness impact profile: Validation of a health status measure. *Medical Care, 14,* 57–67.

Coates, A., Dillenbeck, C. F., McNeil, D. R., Kaye, S. B., Sims, K., Fox, R. M., Woods, R. L., Milton, G. W., Solomon, J., & Tattersall, M. H. (1983). On the receiving end-II. Linear analogue self-assessment (LASA) in evaluation of aspects of the quality of life of cancer patients receiving therapy. *European Journal of Cancer and Clinical Oncology, 19,* 1633–1637.

Daut, R. L., Cleeland, C. S., & Flanery, R. C. (1983). Development of the Wisconsin Brief Pain Questionnaire to assess pain in cancer and other diseases. *Pain, 17,* 197–210.

Derogatis, L. R. (1976). *Scoring and procedures manual for PAIS.* Baltimore, Clinical Psychometric Research.

Derogatis, L. R., & Spencer, P. M. (1984). Psychometric issues in the psychological assessment of the cancer patient. *Cancer, 53,* 2228–2234.

Foley, K. M. (1984). Assessment of pain. In R. G. Twycross (Ed.), *Pain relief in cancer* (pp. 17–31). London: W.B. Saunders Company.

Folstein, M. F., Fetting, A. L., Niaz, U., & Copozzoli, K. D. (1984). Cognitive assessment of cancer patients. *Cancer, 53,* 2250–2255.

Folstein, M., Folstein, S., & McHugh, P. (1975). Mini-mental state: A practical method for grading the cognitive state of patients for the clinician. *Journal of Psychiatry, 12,* 189–198.

Goldfred, M. R., & Lineham, M. M. (1977). Basic issues in behavioral assessment. In A. R. Ciminero, K. S. Calhoun, & H. E. Adams (Eds.) *Handbook of behavioral assessment* (pp. 15–46). New York: John Wiley & Sons.

Gottschalf, L. W. (1984). Measurement of mood and affect in cancer patients. *Cancer, 53,* 2236–2241.

Graham, C., Bond, S. S., Gerkovich, M. M., & Cook, M. R. (1980). Use of the McGill Pain Questionnaire in the assessment of cancer pain: Replicability and consistency. *Pain, 8,* 377–387.

Greenberg, D. B. (1984). The measurement of sexual dysfunction in cancer patients. *Cancer, 53,* 2281–2285.

Henrich, R. L., Schag, C. C., & Ganz, P. A. (1984). Living with cancer: The Cancer Inventory of Problem Situations. *Journal of Clinical Psychology, 40,* 972–980.

Holland, J. C. B. (1976). Coping with cancer: A challenge to the behavioral sciences. In J. W. Cullen, B. H. Fox, & R. N. Jsum (Eds.) *Cancer: The behavioral dimensions.* New York: Raven Press.

Kanfer, F. H., & Saslow, G. (1969). Behavioral diagnosis. In C. M. Franks (Eds.) *Behavior therapy: Appraisal and status.* New York: McGraw-Hill.

Katz, S., & Akpom, C. A. (1966). A measure of primary sociobiological functions. *International Journal of Health Services, 6,* 493–507.

Kent, R. N., & Foster, S. L. (1977). Direct observational procedures: Methodological issues in naturalistic settings. In A. R. Cimenero, K. S. Calhoun, & H. E. Adams (Eds.) *Handbook of behavioral assessment,* (pp. 279–328). New York: John Wiley & Sons.

Mahoney, F. I., & Barthel, D. W. (1965). Functional evaluation: The Barthel Index. *Md State Medical Journal, 14,* 61–65.

Melzack, R. (1975). The McGill Pain Questionnaire: Major properties and scoring methods. *Pain, 1,* 277–299.

Morrow, G. R. (1980). Clinical trials in psychosocial medicine: Methodological and statistical considerations. Part III. Assessing measurement tehcniques in psychosocial oncology. *Cancer Treatment Reports, 64,* 451–456.

Morrow, G. R. (1984). The assessment of nausea and vomiting: Past problems, current issues, and suggestions for future research. *Cancer, 53,* 2267–2278.

Morrow, G. R., Arseneau, J. C., Asbury, R. F., Bennett, J. M., & Boros, L. (1982). Anticipatory nausea and vomiting in chemotherapy patients. *New England Journal of Medicine, 306,* 431–432.

Morrow, G. R., Chiarello, R. J., & Derogatis, L. R. (1978). A new scale for assessing patient's psychosocial adjustment to illness. *Psychological Medicine, 8,* 605–610.

Morrow, G. R., Feldstein, M., Adler, L. M., Derogatis, L. R., Enelow, A. J., Gates, C., Holland, J., Melisarotos, N., Murawski, B. J., Penmari, D., Schmale, A., Schmitt, M., & Morse, J. (1981). Development of brief measures of psychosocial adjustment to medical illness applied to cancer patients. *General Hospital Psychiatry, 3,* 78–88.

McCorkle, R., Packard, N., & Laudenburger, K. (1985). Subject accural and attrition: Problems and solutions. *Journal of Psychosocial Oncology, 2,* 137–146.

Padilla, G. V., Presant, C., Grant, M. M., Metter, G., Lipsett, J., & Heide, F. (1983). Quality of life index for patients with cancer. *Research Nursing Health, 6,* 117–126.

Redd, W. H., Rosenberger, P. H., & Hendler, C. S. (1983). Controlling chemotherapy side effecs. *American Journal of Clinical Hypnosis, 25,* 151–172.

Reitan, R. M. (1955). The relation of the trial making test to organic brain damage. *Journal of Consulting Psychology, 19,* 393–394.

Reitan, R. M. (1958). Validity of the trial making test as an indicator of organic brain damage. *Perception and Motor Skills, 8,* 271–276.

Schnipper, H., Clinch, J., McMurray, A., & Levitt, M. (1984). Measuring the quality of life of cancer patients: The Functional Living Index-Cancer: Development and validation. *Journal of Clinical Oncology, 2,* 472–483.

Silberfarb, P. M. (1984). Response (to Folstein et al., 1984). *Cancer, 53,* 2255–2257.

Sugarbaker, P. H., Barofsky, I., Rosenberg, S. A., & Granola, F. B. (1981). Quality of life assessment of patients in extremity sarcoma clinical trials. *Surgery, 91,* 17–23.

Wallenstein, S. L. (1984). Measurement of pain and analgesia in cancer patients. *Cancer, 53,* 2260–2264.

Wallenstein, S. L., Rogers, A., Kaiko, R. K., Hendrich, G. III, & Houde, R. W. (1980). Relative analgesic potency of oral zomepirac and intramuscular morphine in cancer patients with postoperative pain. *Journal of Clinical Pharmacology, 20,* 250–258.

Weissman, M. W. (1975). The assessment of social adjustment: A review of the techniques. *Archives of General Psychiatry, 32,* 357–365.

Wellisch, D. K. (1984). Work, social, recreation, family, and physical status. *Cancer, 54,* 2290–2299.

Wolff, H. C., & Curran, D. (1955). The nature of delirium and allied states: The dysergastric reaction. *Archives of Neurological Psychiatry. 33,* 1175–1215.

Assessing Pain Among Oncology and Terminally Ill Patients: Psychometric Considerations

Thomas E. Rudy
Dennis C. Turk

ABSTRACT. All too frequently, clinical researchers adopt assessment instruments without considering the psychometric adequacy of the instrument. Although sound research methodology is widely accepted as necessary for the scientific study of pain and its relief, the development and appropriate use of reliable and valid measures of pain is far less appreciated. This paper provides the reader with a basic psychometric primer in order to better evaluate the psychometric properties of pain and other assessment instruments.

At a recent international meeting on cancer, several prominent clinical investigators strongly suggested that pain was not adequately controlled in terminally ill patients. They attributed the poor control to needless fears about narcotic addiction. A critical point that is not made clear by these concerns is how the inadequacy of pain control is determined. The implicit assumption of this statement is that there are satisfactory procedures available to assess pain. In this paper we will discuss how one decides that a specific assessment procedure is adequate. Although we will focus on the assessment of pain, the same psychometric issues and strategies are relevant for all aspects of psychosocial assessment.

Thomas E. Rudy, PhD, is at the Department of Anesthesiology and the Center for Pain Evaluation and Treatment, University of Pittsburgh School of Medicine. Dennis C. Turk, PhD, is at the Department of Psychiatry and the Center for Pain Evaluation and Treatment, University of Pittsburgh School of Medicine.

Support for this paper was provided in part by NIDR grant #1R01DE07514-01.

Requests for reprints should be sent to Thomas E. Rudy, PhD, Center for Pain Evaluation and Treatment, University of Pittsburgh School of Medicine, 230 Lothrop Street, Pittsburgh, PA 15213.

Although sound research methodology is widely accepted as necessary for the scientific study of pain and its relief, the development and appropriate use of reliable and valid measures of pain is far less appreciated. All too often pain measures of unknown psychometric properties are used to assess whether a clinical intervention is effective in relieving or at least reducing an individual's level of pain and the psychosocial disruption caused by pain. Readers of this special issue, regardless of individual discipline or scientific focus, likely hold in common the importance of better understanding pain in cancer and other terminally ill patients and the clinical control of this pain. These objectives, however, cannot be met unless valid, reliable, and flexible measures of pain are utilized.

In this paper we will provide the reader unfamiliar with the basic psychometric principles of reliability and validity with a brief primer. Psychometrics is a branch of psychology devoted to the development of quantitative methods and models for measuring psychological phenomena, including the development of new mathematical and statistical techniques for the evaluation of psychological data and tests. This paper will focus on two major psychometric properties for a test or assessment procedure, reliability and validity. We will also criticize several frequently employed statistical methods that are used by investigators to "demonstrate" the psychometric adequacy of their measures and offer several more acceptable alternatives to these methods. Most importantly, throughout this paper we will emphasize what is the necessary information one needs to know about a pain assessment instrument in order to decide if it is a psychometrically-sound measure that, therefore, may have clinical and/or research utility with terminally ill patients.

SETTING THE STAGE

For the purposes of illustrating basic psychometric principles in the sections that follow, we will use a hypothetical instrument, the Pittsburgh Pain Screening Inventory (i.e., the PPSI) that is designed to assess pain in terminally ill patients. Let us assume that the PPSI adheres to the Melzack-Wall Gate Control Model of pain (1965) in that it acknowledges that pain is a complex, subjective phenomenon that is uniquely experienced by each patient. In other words, this assessment instrument is designed to attend to sensory-discriminative, motivational-affective, and cognitive-evaluative components of the pain experience. That is, cognitive and affective factors are hypothesized to interact with sensory phenomena to create the perception of pain.

To operationalize this conceptualization of pain, we developed the PPSI and created multiple scales that supposedly measure pain severity, negative mood or affective distress due to pain, perceived interference in daily functioning as a result of pain, and patients' perceptions of their ability to control their pain. Additionally, we assert that pain assessment should not be limited to patient's self-report and, therefore, we included in the PPSI a scale to measure "objective" pain behaviors, overt expressions of pain and suffering that can be completed by health-care providers or family members. Finally, we will assume that you are interested in obtaining an instrument that measures pain in oncology patients in order to assess whether your interventions are effective in controlling their pain and decide to write to us for a copy of the PPSI and a user's manual. However, being a skeptical consumer of research you want to evaluate the psychometric adequacy of the PPSI before you begin to use it with your patients. How would you go about conducting this evaluation? Below are some of the basic psychometric criteria you should apply to the PPSI before you conclude that this instrument meets the necessary scientific standards to truly be a satisfactory measure of pain.

RELIABILITY

The first question you should ask about the PPSI is whether it is reliable. Reliability concerns the extent to which a test or for that matter any measuring procedure yields the same results on repeated trials. Nunally (1978) has defined reliability as follows:

> Reliability concerns the extent to which measurements are repeatable—when different persons make the measurements, on different occasions, with supposedly alter-

native instruments for measuring the same thing and when there are small variations in circumstances for making measurements that are not intended to influence results. In other words, measurements are intended to be stable over a variety of conditions in which essentially the same results should be obtained. (p. 191)

It should be noted that the measurement of any phenomenon, including an individual's experience of pain, always contains a certain amount of chance variation. The goal of error-free measurement, while an important goal to strive for, is never attained in any area of science. As Stanley (1971) points out, "the discrepancies between two sets of measurements may be expressed in miles and, in other cases, in millionths of a millimeter; but, if the unit of measurement is fine enough in relation to the accuracy of the measurements, discrepancies always will appear" (p. 356). This implies that two sets of measurements of the same features on the same individual will never exactly duplicate each other. For example, a blood sample may be drawn from an individual and half of it sent to a laboratory for a chemical profile analysis and the other half is not sent to the same laboratory until next day. The agreement between the two analyses of the same blood sample is an indication of the reliability of the chemical profile analysis. The two laboratory analyses, however, will not be in perfect agreement because numerous sources of error can affect these measures (e.g., the laboratory may have recalibrated their equipment between the two analyses, two different technicians conducted the analyses, etc.).

For the PPSI to be considered a reliable pain assessment instrument it should generally contain small errors of measurement. In other words, its scales should show stability, consistency, and dependability. The more reliable the PPSI scales are, the more consistent or stable they should be over repeated measurements provided that no treatment interventions or other unusual events have occurred between these measurements.

Methods of Assessing Reliability

When you read the user's manual for the PPSI, you should note whether some type of reliability coefficient is reported for each of the PPSI scales. You should also be aware, however, that the term reliability coefficient is a generic term and can be computed in a number of different ways.

Test-Retest Method

One of the easiest and most frequently used ways to estimate the reliability of a measure or scale is by the test-retest method. For example, the reliability of the pain severity scale on the PPSI may have been established by administering this scale to a group of oncology patients at one point in time and then readministering this same scale to the same group of patients at a later point in time. The reliability of the PPSI's pain severity scale can then be computed by correlating the two sets of patients' pain severity scores.

Although the test-retest method seems to yield one of the most reasonable estimates of the reliability of a measure (Allen & Yen, 1979), there are several complications inherent with this method. Perhaps the most serious complication is the potential for reactivity or a carry-over effect between assessments; that is, the results of the first assessment may influence the results obtained in the second assessment. For example, the patient may simply remember his or her answers on the PPSI's pain severity scale from the first administration and repeat them at the second time of testing.

An additional problem with the test-retest method involves the length of time between the two test administrations. A very short time interval may encourage carry-over effects due to memory and lead to an inflated reliability estimate, while a very long time may lead to an underestimation of the true reliability of a measure. For example, to administer the PPSI's pain severity measure to oncology patients who are in intense pain and then wait for a month to readminister this measure would likely lead to an inaccurate estimate of the scale's reliability because most of these individuals would have received some form of treatment for their pain during the month separating the two measures of pain severity. At least for individuals with chronic, benign pain, we (Kerns, Turk, & Rudy, 1985) have found one to two weeks between pain assessments to be a sufficient time to establish the test-retest reliability of pain measures. This time interval is frequently the time period recommended for assessing the reliability of other types of measures (e.g., Nunally, 1964).

Alternative-Form Method

Although the developers of the PPSI may fail to report test-retest reliability for a scale, another acceptable method for establishing scale reliability is the alternative-form method. This approach to reliability is similar to the test-retest method in that it also requires two testing situations with the same individuals. However, rather than simply administering the same test on the second testing occasion, the developers may create an alternate test form of a scale in such a way that its content parallels that of the first form of the scale. For example, we may create two different but equivalent scales to assess affective distress due to pain and then administer these separate scales to the same patients at two points in time. The correlation between these two alternative forms of affective distress is then used as an estimate of the reliability of the scale. In general, this method is superior to the simple test-retest method because it reduces the extent to which individuals' memory can inflate the reliability estimate. A limitation of this method, however, is that it is often difficult to construct two alternative forms that are indeed parallel to each other in content.

Internal-Consistency

The authors of the PPSI report that several of its scales are comprised of multiple items that are summed to yield a scale score. For example, the PPSI scale designed to measure pain interference with daily functioning may contain multiple questions related to how pain interferes with the individual's sleep, how it interferes with the ability to perform household chores, how it interferes with family and social relationships, and so forth. The authors of the PPSI should provide evidence that the summed items on the interference scale, indeed, are highly interrelated. This is usually accomplished by calculating an internal-consistency estimate of reliability. This reliability coefficient can be computed by using only one test administration and, as such, avoid the problems associated with repeated testings. The most frequently used internal-consistency reliability estimate is Cronbach's alpha (Cronbach, 1951). If all the items in a scale are highly intercorrelated the scale will demonstrate high internal agreement or consistency among the items of the scale. Internal consistency is usually reported as "coefficient alpha" (basically the average correlation among the items in the scale).

Thus, internal-consistency reliability measures are designed to assess whether a group of items are homogeneous. If so, a more reliable scale can usually be created by summing these items, that is, multiple-item scales are usually much more reliable than a single-item scale. For example, asking a patient to rate their pain intensity on a single-item scale ranging from 0 = none to 3 = severe, will not be as reliable as a scale consisting of several items related to pain severity. Thus, having patients rate their present pain intensity, the amount of pain that they have experienced in the last hour, and the amount of suffering caused by this pain and then summing these three items would create a more reliable measure of pain intensity. It should be noted, however, that reliability coefficients based on internal analyses should not be interpreted as substitutes for alternate-form reliability or as estimates of the stability of a scale over time.

Inter-Rater Reliability

As you recall, the authors of the PPSI included a scale designed to measure pain behaviors that is to be completed by persons other than the patient. Although recognizing that pain is ultimately a subjective, personal experience, the authors of the PPSI assert that there are certain behaviors that can be observed by others and used as indicators of pain. Seven pain behaviors are included in the PPSI and include items such as verbal complaints of pain, nonverbal complaints of pain (e.g., moans and groans), facial grimaces, and clutching or rubbing the site of pain. A 3-point scale, comprised of none, occasionally, and frequently, is provided with each pain behavior and the observer is asked to rate the frequency of occurrence of each of these behaviors for a particular patient. From a reliability standpoint, the question is whether multiple observers of the same patient can agree on the frequency of each of the seven pain behaviors contained in the PPSI. What evidence would you need to be convinced that the PPSI pain behavior scale is reliable?

If we reported that the sum of these pain behaviors for 30 patients had a high correlation between two independent raters, would you conclude that the pain behaviors scale is reliable? Hopefully not. Although frequently used to establish inter-rater reliability, the correlation coefficient is not an appropriate statistic to demonstrate inter-rater reliability (Bartko & Carpenter, 1976). For example, it is possible for the correlation between two raters to be perfect yet they actually disagree in their ratings.

If we reported that two independent raters showed an average of 80% agreement in rating each of the PPSI pain behaviors, could one conclude that the PPSI pain behavior scale is reliable? The percentage of agreement among independent raters, computed by taking the total number of inter-rater agreements and dividing this number by the total number of possible ratings, is also not an acceptable method of computing inter-rater reliability. This method does not take chance agreement into account and there are no statistical tests of significance; that is, there is no way to statistically determine what percentage is high enough to be acceptable. Two better methods of establishing inter-rater reliability would be to compute either a weighted kappa coefficient or an intraclass correlation. Both of these methods adjusts for chance agreement and provide a statistical test of significance (see Bartko & Carpenter, 1976 for methods that can be used to calculate these reliability coefficients).

How Good is Good?

A frequent difficulty in evaluating the psychometric adequacy of a scale is deciding what is an acceptable level of reliability. As is often done, we may conclude our discussion of the PPSI's reliability coefficients with the phrase " . . . thus all PPSI scales displayed good reliability." Unfortunately, it is not easy to specify a single level to indicate a satisfactory level of reliability. One reasonable set of guidelines for interpreting reliability coefficients is provided by Cicchetti and Sparrow (1981). These authors suggest that any reliability value less than .40 be considered poor, values between .40 and .59 are fair, values between .60 and .74 are good, and reliability coefficients .75 or over are excellent.

No matter what reliability criterion you accept as adequate for your purposes, you should be aware that scales with lower reliability may not perform in predictable or dependable ways. For example, you may want to measure the effectiveness of an analgesic drug intervention for a group of cancer patients experiencing severe pain and decide to use the PPSI pain severity scale as your measure of treatment change. If this scale is not very reliable and you find that your treatment intervention did not produce significant pre-post changes in pain severity, you cannot be sure whether this nonsignificant effect was due to your treatment or the large amount of measurement error (i.e., low reliability) contained within the pain severity scale.

VALIDITY

After using the above information in your evaluation of the PPSI, you may conclude that the reliability of this instrument was adequately developed and all the scales of the PPSI had satisfactory levels of reliability. A second and perhaps more important consideration in your evaluation of the PPSI is whether it is a valid instrument; does the instrument measure what it purports to measure? Stated differently, validity refers to the appropriateness, meaningfulness, and usefulness of the specific inferences made from the scores obtained from a test. The validity of a test is often a matter of degree and can be established by a multitude of methods. Below we will review three of the most important types of validity: content validity, criterion-related validity, and construct validity.

Content Validity

Content validity is usually established through a rational analysis of the content of a test and its determination is basically the result of an individual, subjective judgment (Allen & Yen, 1979). Although subjective, its importance should not be minimized nor is it as simple a process as it might appear. Primarily, content validity is concerned with determining whether a scale or test has sufficient content to adequately cover or represent the domain a test purports to measure. For example, if the PPSI pain behavior scale only contained one item (e.g., facial grimacing), we might conclude the domain of pain behaviors was not sampled with sufficient breadth to truly represent a measure of pain behaviors.

Criterion-Related Validity

Criterion-related validity indicates the effectiveness of a test in predicting an individual's behavior in specified situations. In other words, criterion-related evidence demonstrates that test scores are systematically related to one or more outcome criteria. Naturally, the choice of the criterion and how it is measured is of central importance in determining criterion-related validity. In terms of the PPSI scales, we would hope that measures of pain severity and the amount of perceived life interference due to pain would be predictive of staff observed activity levels, participation in family activities, degree of pain behaviors, and so forth. Additionally, the PPSI scale that measures to what degree patients feel they are able to control their pain should be predictive of the amount and frequency of medication usage. Although very few developers of pain assessment scales report evidence for criterion-related validity, this instrument quality becomes important if a measure is to be used diagnostically or for clinical decision making.

Construct Validity

Construct validity is a more recently developed form of validity and refers to the degree to which a test or scale measures the theoretical construct or concept that it was designed to measure. Construct validity becomes particularly important to establish when we attempt to measure abstract concepts, of which pain is one. That is, because there are no objective yardsticks by which to measure pain, the validity of our measures of pain can only be established indirectly.

Documenting the construct validity of a measure is an ongoing process and is often based on the test developer making predictions about how a scale or assessment technique should behave in various situations. These predictions can then be tested and, if the predictions are supported by the data, the evidence of construct validity is enhanced. For example, to demonstrate the validity of the PPSI scale used to measure negative mood or affective distress we might hypothesize that this scale should be positively correlated with another mood measure that has already been demonstrated to have adequate psychometric properties. To test this prediction, we might administer these two scales to a group of patients who are experiencing at least some pain and compute the correlation between the two scales. If the correlation was positive and significant, this would provide preliminary evidence for the construct validity of the PPSI negative mood scale.

Another method to demonstrate construct validity is to conduct an experimental intervention that theoretically should produce a change in the scale under question. For example, we may use the PPSI pain severity scale before and after an analgesic intervention and would expect a significant reduction in pain severity scores. If a significant decrease is not found, although we would not immediately discard the pain severity scale because factors other than poor scale validity may have been at work in this experiment, we would begin to question whether this scale does indeed measure the construct of pain severity.

THE AVAILABILITY OF NORMS

In the absence of normative information, a raw score on any test is meaningless. To say that a patient with cancer of the pancreas has a score of 10 on the PPSI pain severity scale conveys little or no information. However, if you know that the average pain severity value for 30 patients with pancreatic cancer was 5.4 with a standard deviation of 1.1, you would conclude that this particular patient is expressing a particularly high level of pain.

This example highlights the importance of having normative information about a test, preferably on the type of population with which you intend to use the test. The minimal amount of normative information the test developer should provide you with is the mean and standard deviation for each scale on a test and, if a test has multiple scales, the intercorrelations among the scales. Additionally, you should know for what population(s) norms are available. For example, if we developed the PPSI by using 100 head and neck patients and you want to use the PPSI with a group of patients with leukemia, this does not necessary mean that the PPSI is inappropriate for your use but it does mean that the norms that we developed are not likely to be appropriate for your particular cancer population. In general, it is preferable to use an instrument for which norms are already established for the particular population you wish to use it with. However, it should be recognized that establishing norms for many different populations is extremely difficult and costly. You may need to choose an instrument that has well established reliability and construct validity, and then use it for some time with your particular population and develop your own norms.

SUMMING UP

It is all too often the case that a newly published assessment instrument is adopted by clinical researchers without considering the important psychometric issues that we have described. Conclusions such as those reached by the clinical investigators on the adequate use of narcotics for pain control in the terminally ill are predicated on the adequacy of the assessment instrument employed. We need to first ask *how* was pain control or relief measured and *if* the conclusion is warranted based on the assessment strategy.

An instrument may sound like "just what you've been looking for," but careful consideration of the psychometric adequacy of that instrument should be addressed before adopting it. Although we have used assessment of pain to illustrate some of the relevant issues to be considered in selecting an assessment instrument, the psychometric considerations outlined are relevant for assessing any psychosocial instrument.

REFERENCES

Allen, M.J., & Yen, W.M. (1979). *Introduction to measurement theory.* Monterey, CA: Brooks/Cole Publishing.

Anastasi, A. (1968). *Psychological testing* (3rd ed.). New York: MacMillan.

Bartko, J.J., & Carpenter, W.T. (1976). On the methods and theory of reliability. *The Journal of Nervous and Mental Disease, 163,* 307–317.

Cicchetti, D.V., & Sparrow, S.S. (1981). Developing criteria for establishing inter-rater reliability of specific items: Applications to assessment of adaptive behavior. *American Journal of Mental Deficiency, 86,* 127–137.

Cronbach, L.J. (1951). Coefficient alpha and the internal structure of tests. *Psychometrika, 16,* 297–334.

Kerns, R.D., Turk, D.C., & Rudy, T.E. (1985). The West Haven-Yale Multidimensional Pain Inventory (WHYMPI). *Pain, 23,* 345–356.

Melzack, R., & Wall, P.D. (1965). Pain mechanisms: A new theory. *Science, 50,* 971–979.

Nunally, J.C. (1964). *Educational measurement and evaluation.* New York: McGraw-Hill.

Nunally, J.C. (1978). *Psychometric theory* (2nd ed.). New York: McGraw-Hill.

Stanley, J.C. (1971). Reliability. In R.L. Thorndike (Ed.), *Educational measurement* pp. 356–442. Washington, DC: American Council on Education.

Assessment of Acute Pain and Anxiety and Chemotherapy-Related Nausea and Vomiting in Children and Adolescents

Lonnie Zeltzer
Samuel LeBaron

ABSTRACT. Assessment of pain, anxiety, nausea, and vomiting in children and adolescents has some unique features which require special consideration. Developmental needs are outlined and data on assessment of pain and anxiety in infants, children, and adolescents are reviewed. Specifically, behavioral, physiological, and self-assessment methods are summarized and critiqued. The interrelationships between these methods are discussed, while a focus on the clinical meaning of these data is maintained. The limited data on nausea and vomiting in children receiving chemotherapy are also reviewed. Recommendations are made regarding the clinical usefulness of assessment methods for pain, anxiety, nausea, and vomiting in children, while areas of controversy are pointed out.

Many catastrophic childhood illnesses of yesterday have become the chronic diseases of today's children and adolescents. Newer, more powerful drugs, combined with better diagnostic modalities, have increased survival rates, but have also in-

We wish to thank Miss Jo Ann Lieberman for her help in preparation of this manuscript. This investigation was supported by PHS Grant Numbers 5 R01 CA36101 (Doctors Zeltzer and LeBaron) and 1 K04 CA00938 (RCDA, Doctor Zeltzer), awarded by the National Cancer Institute, DHHS; and by the W. T. Grant Foundation Faculty Scholars Program (Doctor Zeltzer).

Lonnie Zeltzer, MD and Samuel LeBaron, PhD; Associates Professors; Division of Adolescent Medicine; Department of Pediatrics; The University of Texas Health Science Center at San Antonio; 7703 Floyd Curl Drive; San Antonio, TX 78284-7803.

creased side effects and invasiveness of treatment. With the increase in survival rates, some investigators have looked for ways to improve the quality of life for these children and adolescents. These investigations have led to the development of a technology for assessing qualitative aspects of treatment, such as pain, nausea, or acute anxiety. The purpose of this paper is to review the unique issues related to assessment of distressing symptoms that interfere with children's quality of life. This review will focus on acute pain and anxiety and chemotherapy-related nausea and vomiting, since these seem to be the most troublesome for children. These symptoms have been the focus for the majority of pharmacological and behavioral intervention studies in sick children and adolescents, especially those with cancer.

GENERAL DEVELOPMENTAL CONSIDERATIONS

What is unique about children? Why do we not simply transfer the assessment methods used in studies of adults to children? The most important reason is that there are basic differences between children and adults in cognitive development and life experience. Such differences can affect how a symptom is perceived, and how that perception and experience of the symptom are communicated to others.

Because children have relatively less experience, conceptual ability, and social maturity than adults, their understanding of and communication about symptoms is often limited. The ability to distinguish one symptom from another is crucial in most research in this area. Most adults seem to have a clearer understanding than do children of the difference between pain and anxiety, for example. Schultz (1971) questioned 74 children, ages 10 and 11 years, about pain. It was found that 84% related pain to anxiety ("being afraid") and almost all of the children related pain to bodily injury and death. Such feelings may become mixed together in descriptions. In fact, some investigators *prefer* to combine assessment of pain and anxiety into a single measure of "distress," usually based on observations of children's behaviors.

Many young children have not yet developed enough vocabulary and conceptual ability to describe symptoms accurately and to categorize various degrees of distress. Another problem in the assessment of children is that their perceptions of a symptom such as pain or nausea are very malleable. The separation from parents and the unfamiliarity with the medical setting and medical procedures can produce such a degree of anxiety that some children experience a relatively minor pain (e.g., a finger prick) as a major source of discomfort.

Most adults are able to describe, rate, or otherwise respond to requests of strangers in a medical setting when asked about their symptoms. Because children are less mature socially, they are less likely to talk candidly about their problems to a stranger. Unless the child feels secure, his/her responses appear more likely than adults to reflect social compliance rather than a genuine and valid report of symptoms. In a study of 994 children (5–12 years), Ross and Ross (1984) found that the type of questions asked, the climate of the interview, and the relationship between the child and the interviewer all significantly affected the child's responses about his/her symptoms.

ASSESSMENT OF PAIN AND ANXIETY

Assessment of Infants

The investigation of pain in infants has focused primarily on infant cries. Wasz-Hockert, Lind, Vuorenkoski, Partanen, and Valanne (1968) examined the acoustical properties of infant cries and found that pain cries were less likely than other cries to have rising/falling characteristics and were more likely to last longer. In two studies of tape recordings of infants (Wolfe, 1969; Zeskind, Sale, Maio, Huntington, & Weiseman, 1985), the initial portion of cries was found to be the segment which elicited adult attention and presumably communicated a heightened level of infant arousal. In a review of studies analyzing the cries of human infants and primates, Levine and Gordon (1982) found pain cries to be unique and unlike the cries of hunger and other sensations.

In addition to cries, behavioral and physiological assessments have also been made in infants. Craig, McMahon, Morison, and Zaskow (1984) examined developmental changes in pain expression provoked by routine immunization injections in infants under two years of age. Infants less than 12 months of age responded to injections in an apparently random, diffuse manner, whereas infants 12–24 months of age displayed more anticipatory distress, descriptive language, and goal directed movement. Unfortunately, the relationship between infants' cries and their behavior was not assessed. Palmar sweating during heel pricks was found in newborns over 37 weeks gestation (Harper & Rutter, 1982). While it may be assumed that this physiological parameter indicated pain in the neonates, no other measures were used (e.g., infant cries) to corroborate this belief.

In summary, infants demonstrate their distress associated with pain through changes in the nature of their cries. As they approach toddlerhood, they are able to contribute more demonstrable language and body movements to indicate pain. Physiological indices of pain in infants have not yet been validated against cries or pain-associated behaviors. Other such behaviors of longer duration, such as sleep or feeding disturbances, also warrant investigation for a fuller understanding of the nature of pain in infants.

Assessment of Children and Adolescents

Behavioral Assessment

Behavioral assessment of pain and anxiety in children and adolescents has followed two formats. One approach is to observe and list the child's behaviors during a painful medical or dental procedure. Behavioral checklists have been used to help standardize the observations. These behavioral checklists are presumed by some investigators to measure a construct most commonly called "distress," which has been described as consisting of a combination of pain and anxiety (Katz, Varni, & Jay, 1984). The second assessment format has been observers' global estimates (expressed numerically as ratings) of the extent of the child's pain and anxiety during a particular painful procedure or period of time.

The first systematic use of a behavioral checklist was reported by Katz, Kellerman, and Siegel (1980) in an assessment study of 77 patients (2 to 16 years) undergoing bone marrow aspirations (BMA's). Observers used a 13-item behavioral checklist and made global observational ratings of distress. Children 10 years of age or less appeared, on the basis of their behavior, to be more "distressed" during bone marrow aspirations than were adolescents. The greatest variety of "stress-related" behaviors (i.e., an undifferentiated pattern of crying, protesting, and resistance) occurred in children younger than 6 years of age. Sacham and Daut (1981) questioned the validity of measuring "distress" and proposed that both pain *and* anxiety should be assessed in children. Katz, Kellerman, and Siegel (1981) argued that separate assessment of pain and anxiety is difficult in children, and that a combination, which they called "distress," is probably the most useful construct for identifying those children who need intervention.

Two groups of investigators developed modifications of the behavioral checklist format. In a study of 50 children and adolescents undergoing BMA's, LeBaron and Zeltzer (1984) used an 8-item behavioral checklist, observer ratings of pain and anxiety, and children's self-reports of pain and anxiety. This study seemed to replicate the finding of Katz et al. (1980); children showed more "distress" behaviors compared to adolescents. However, with the inclusion of two additional behaviors seen primarily in adolescents (i.e., flinching and groaning), these age differences were eliminated. These results suggested that both checklists, as they were originally designed, were age-biased. No age, sex, or ethnic differences were found for the enlarged behavioral checklist. The checklist by LeBaron and Zeltzer (1984) also included ratings (0–10 scale) of the intensity of each behavior observed. These intensity ratings did not distinguish between children and adolescents. When behaviors occurred, they were usually rated as intense, regardless of age.

Jay, Ozolins, Elliott, and Caldwell (1983) reported a modification of the Katz checklist in which each item was weighted. A priori, each of the behaviors on the checklist was assigned a "severity-of-distress" value (1–4 scale) by three clinic staff familiar with bone marrow aspirations. Also, behavioral ratings using the checklist were made at 15-second intervals during the medical procedure rather than at three categorical procedure-related intervals (immediately before, during, and after) as in the studies by Katz et al. (1980) and LeBaron and Zeltzer (1984). Correlations between the modified checklist (i.e., "weighted" behaviors and frequent assessments) and children's ratings of pain or observers' ratings of "distress" were not significantly higher than correlations made for the checklist without these modifications (Jay & Elliott, 1984). The apparent age-bias in the checklists used by Katz et al. (1980) and LeBaron and Zeltzer (1984) was also replicated. That is, children displayed more of the behaviors on the original and modified checklists than did adolescents.

Ratings based on observers' global assessments of children's pain and anxiety have been used primarily in behavioral intervention studies of children undergoing painful procedures. These observers' ratings have been based typically on Likert scales of varying expansion (Hilgard & LeBaron, 1982; Jay et al., 1983; Katz et al., 1980; Kellerman et al., 1983; Zeltzer & LeBaron, 1982). The observers have been either trained research assistants (Hilgard & LeBaron, 1982; LeBaron & Zeltzer, 1984; Zeltzer & LeBaron, 1982), nurses (Jay & Elliott, 1984; Jay, Elliott, Katz, & Siegel, 1985; Jay et al., 1983; Katz et al., 1980 and submitted), or parents (Jay & Elliott, 1984; Jay et al., 1985). The relationship of the observer to the child may play a role in the objectivity of the observations. For example, correlations between a behavioral checklist and parent ratings of distress ($r = .38$) (Jay et al., 1983) were much lower than between the checklist and nurses' ratings ($r = .73$) (Jay & Elliott, 1984).

Physiological Assessment

Physiological measures have been used in only a few studies. In a study to validate a behavioral checklist, Jay and Elliott (1984) measured heart rate at three different time periods (at clinic entry, upon entering the treatment room, and after completion of the medical procedure). As part of a behavioral intervention study, Jay et al. (1985) assessed heart rate, blood pressure, and palmar sweat during the above time periods in children undergoing bone marrow aspirations. In a personal communication, Jay reported that, compared to assessment of heart rate and blood pressure, measurements of palmar sweat were time-consuming, difficult to accomplish, and did not seem to produce data which added significantly to an understanding of the patients' experience. Abu-Saad (1981) assessed pulse, temperature, respiratory rate, and blood pressure in 10 children during the first two days following surgery. However, while mean values for these physiological parameters are given in her study, no analyses of the data are provided. The question of the meaning of physiological data in studies of children's pain and anxiety is an important one and will be discussed in more depth later in the section on the clinical meaning of assessment.

Children's Self-Assessment

A variety of instruments have been used to measure children's self-reports of their own pain and anxiety. The most simple of these have been numerical ratings or variations of a visual analog scale. Hilgard and LeBaron used a 10-point Likert scale for children to rate their pain during bone marrow aspirations (1982). They included faces depicting increasing amounts of "distress" as guideposts on the numerical rating scale. They also permitted the children to use a number "greater than 10" if the child felt the need to do so (Hilgard & LeBaron, 1984). A similar five-point Likert scale with accompanying faces was used by LeBaron and Zeltzer (1984) and Zeltzer and LeBaron (1982) for children's ratings of both pain and anxiety during bone marrow aspirations and lumbar punctures. A five-point numerical scale without faces was used for adolescents' ratings of pain and anxiety by Kellerman et al. (1983). Katz et al. (submitted) used seven faces ranging from smiling to sad to assess self-reports of anxiety (these were called "fear faces"). A review of self-report measures of children's anxiety, primarily in dental settings, can be found in Winer (1982). However, in none of the above studies or in those described below have the rating scales themselves been assessed for developmental validity. That is, what ability do children have, at various developmental stages, to understand and accurately use a particular symptom rating scale?

Variations on the visual analog scale for children's self-assessment of pain have been used by Abu-Saad (a 10 cm line) (1981) and by Katz (a "pain thermometer") (submitted). A series of "visual analog toys" are described (but not assessed)

by White and Stow (1985). The use of colors to depict children's self-reports of pain has been described primarily by
Eland (Eland & Anderson, 1977). While the development of
her color tool has been referred to in several chapters (Jeans,
1983; Eland & Anderson, 1977), reliability and validity data on
the instrument have not been published (i.e., references
include several unpublished masters' theses in Eland and Anderson, 1977 and Eland, 1981). This is unfortunate, since a
number of investigators are using the color tool, with various
modifications, as the primary instrument to test efficacy of
intervention strategies. For example, in a study of intervention
for intramuscular injection pain, Eland (1981) uses an adaptation of her color tool based on two unpublished masters' theses
from the Universities of Washington and Cincinnati. In this
adaptation, the child is asked to select four colors among eight
to represent four gradations of pain from worst to least. Presumably, these four colors are remembered by the child and will
consistently represent the same gradations of pain for the duration of a given study. However, evidence of this has not been
documented.

Eland (Eland & Anderson, 1977) described red, black, and
purple as being the most common colors children use to depict pain. The only published documentation of color prefer-
ence was found in a study by Jeans (1983). In her study,
children were given five markers in colors of blue, black, red,
yellow, and green, and were asked to draw a picture representative of pain. For this task, almost 95% of the group
chose red and/or black. However, how colors relate to gradations of pain is less clear. Based on Eland's unpublished
work, Lollar, Smits, and Patterson (1982) selected the colors
red, yellow, and green to represent much, some, and a little
pain. This self-report measure was then used to develop and
evaluate a projective, trait-related instrument designed to assess children's perceptions of pain. This instrument consisted
of 24 pictures depicting pain situations in four different settings. The child was asked to use the three colors to answer a
series of questions about these pictures. Given the lack of
published data on this use of colors, there is difficulty in
interpreting the age differences found and the significant differences noted between child and parent ratings of pain in the
study by Lollar et al. (1982).

The ability of children to communicate with others about their pain has also been studied. Ross and Ross (1984a) interviewed 994 children ages 5 to 12 years. They found that children can use a variety of adjectives to describe their pain; most define it as general discomfort (e.g., "Pain is when it hurts"). Few mentioned the process or function of pain. Most children emphasized negative aspects of pain.

Interrelationships Between Observational, Physiological, and Self-Report Measures

The relationships between behavioral observations, physiological assessments, and children's self-reports have been studied in various combinations. Behavioral checklist scores have consistently correlated more highly with observers' ratings than with children's self-ratings of pain and anxiety (Jay & Elliott, 1984; Jay et al., 1985; Jay et al., 1983; Katz et al., submitted; LeBaron & Zeltzer, 1984). This relationship makes sense if one assumes that the observer uses the child's behaviors during a procedure as a major factor in making a global assessment. Observer ratings also apparently take into account some qualitative aspects of behavior, since observers' global ratings of pain and anxiety have correlated more highly with children's ratings than have behavioral checklists (Jay & Elliott, 1985; Jay et al., 1985; Jay et al., 1983; Katz et al., submitted; LeBaron & Zeltzer, 1984). The observer's intuitive ability to synthesize objectively definable behaviors and more subtle qualitative factors suggests that a well-trained observer can make a suprisingly valid estimate of children's pain and anxiety, at least for some patients. However, confounding factors such as the age of the patient make the observer's task much more difficult. For example, Hilgard and LeBaron (1982) found significant differences between observers' ratings and adolescents' self-ratings of pain, but no difference for younger children. A similar age relationship was found by Katz et al. (1980) and Jay et al. (1983) for both behavioral checklist scores and observational ratings. Apparently, children have less control over their behaviors than do adolescents, who tend to suffer more privately. Thus, the older the child, the more difficulty the observer has in estimating the patient's pain and anxiety. Both behavioral checklist and observational ratings correlate more highly with children's ratings of anxiety than with children's pain ratings (Katz et al., submitted; LeBaron & Zeltzer, 1984). Perhaps children's anxiety is displayed more readily through their body movements, crying, and stalling tactics, while their private suffering cannot be fully understood unless the child is asked about it.

Correlations between physiological measures and behavioral ratings or self-reports have been inconsistent. Jay and colleagues found that heart rate just prior to bone marrow aspirations correlated quite strongly with behavioral checklist scores (r = .60) (Jay & Elliott, 1986) and with nurses' ratings of children's "distress" (r = .69) (Jay et al., 1986). The correlation between heart rate and children's "fear" ratings was lower (r = .38), and there was no significant relationship between heart rate and children's pain ratings (Jay et al., 1986). Diastolic blood pressure just prior to the procedure was correlated only with the behavioral checklist (r = .38), and palmar sweat showed no appreciable relationship with other parameters (Jay et al., 1986). Heart rate and blood pressure correlated moderately well (r ranged between .40 and .47) with each other. Abu-Saad (1981) found no relationship between children's self-ratings of pain and measures of temperature, heart rate, respiratory rate, or blood pressure. In summary, strong relationships between physiological measures and self- or observer reports have not been found, except for the relationship between pulse and observer measures in one study (Jay et al., 1986).

The Clinical Meaning of Assessments

If one type of observational assessment correlates highly with another but less so with children's self-assessments and not at all with physiological measures, then what is being assessed? As Sacham and Daut (1981) have pointed out, and as LeBaron and Zeltzer (1984) have shown, observational measures assess how the child behaves when experiencing differing combinations of pain and anxiety. Some investigators (Jay et al. 1983; Katz et al., 1980) have labeled this construct "distress." This approach is defensible in view of the difficulty in separating pain and anxiety. For any patient, but for children especially, there are some instances in which the experiences of pain and anxiety seem to be very distinct, and others in which they appear to be indistinguishable. However, the pain and anxiety components of distress may differ among children (or perhaps even situationally for the same child). Thus, behavioral measures when used in isolation do not tell the investigator the extent to which the child's behavior is modulated by pain versus anxiety. With cognitive maturity, older children and adolescents are able to muster some control over their anxiety (and global body movements). Thus, they *appear* to be in less distress than are children during medical procedures, as found in studies by Katz et al. (1980) and Jay et al. (1983).

The best way to find out differentially about children's pain and anxiety is to ask them. The validity of the variety of self-assessment instruments (e.g., numerical scales with or without accompanying faces, visual analog scales, or the use of colors as symbols for extent of pain) has not been adequately assessed. At what age can children reliably use such instruments to communicate their experience of pain and anxiety? Neither a developmental assessment of such self-rating instruments nor a comparison of the instruments to each other has been performed.

Even if the child has a good relationship with the interviewer, can the child's self-report be believed? While searching for ways to validate observational and self-report data, some investigators have turned to physiological measures in hopes of "objectifying" children's experience of pain and/or anxiety. However, the meaning of physiological findings in behavioral studies remains unclear. Often, changes in these variables (e.g., systolic blood pressure reduction from 104 to 99 with intervention) may be statistically significant, but not clinically meaningful. What do elevated heart rate and mildly elevated (but still normal) blood pressure in a screaming child indicate? Do they provide further evidence of "arousal" or is observation of the child sufficient? If physiological assessments are to be made, then it is the job of the investigator to discuss hypotheses about their significance so that these hypotheses can be tested.

Which measure then is real? Can children be anxious without documented physiological arousal? What is the relationship between pain and physiological arousal if there is a relatively low anxiety component? Part of the reason for the inconsistent findings may lie in the lability of children's pulse, respiratory rate, and blood pressure from the moment children enter a medical setting (especially if they have had previous negative experiences in that setting) until they leave. That is, the baseline fluctuations in these physiological variables for children are not known. For example, what effect does suggestion (positive or negative) have on these parameters? Also, some children may be more rapid and extensive adrenergic responders than others with the same experience of pain/anxiety. Basic research in the laboratory setting is needed to answer these questions before physiological indices can be used as outcome measures.

Given the above considerations and confusion, we need to re-ask the question, "What are we assessing?" Perhaps the simplest answer is that each assessment modality is measuring a different component of the child's experience of pain and anxiety. All components are likely interrelated to varying degrees which may differ both individually and situationally. The decision to assess any or all components depends upon why the assessment is being made. Usually the goals of assessment are (a) to identify those children in need of intervention to mitigate their suffering and then (b) to evaluate the efficacy of the intervention. For example, in a clinical situation a psychologist might be consulted to help a child to cope with a medical procedure. Behavioral observation finds a screaming child and tense staff. One goal might be to reduce the child's behavioral distress, thereby also reducing the staff's anxiety and enhancing their feelings of appreciation for the psychologist. However, suppose that the child reports little pain and anxiety and informs the psychologist that screaming helps him to cope effectively with the procedure. The psychologist needs to select the goals of intervention and methods of determining efficacy.

Such children are found in studies of behavioral intervention. Observational data, if used alone, might suggest lack of efficacy of the intervention. Self-report data would give information about the child's personal experience, but may say more about the subjects than about the intervention.

On the other hand, a behavioral strategy may in fact be effective in altering children's behaviors during medical procedures. By observational criteria the intervention is a success.

However, self-report data might indicate that children's private suffering remained unchanged or reduced only slightly. Is the intervention effective or is it not? By the medical staff's criteria, the intervention is a success because the children are more manageable and the clinic may run more efficiently. Additionally, a quieter, happier clinic environment (i.e., less screaming from formerly resistant children) may help to reduce the anxiety of other children about to have medical procedures. But, what is the effect of lowered behaviorally *observed* distress on children who *continue* to report moderate or severe pain and/or anxiety? While we interviewed children in our studies after each procedure and also inquired of parents about any longer-term sequelae of procedure-related suffering, neither we nor anyone else have reported the findings of systematically acquired information of this type. Such follow-up data would be a critical adjunct to on-line assessment in determining efficacy of intervention. Information could be sought about sleep disturbance, behavioral changes, school attendance, etc.

Another example of problems in determining which assessment instruments to choose in evaluating an intervention strategy comes from a study of behavioral intervention for bone marrow aspirations in children 6–10 years of age (Katz et al., submitted). In this study, a reduction in children's self-reports of pain and anxiety was found, but there was no corresponding reduction seen in behavioral measures. Which of the two assessment modalities measured the "efficacy" of the intervention? One possible explanation for the finding is that these young children were unable to control their bodies and verbal expressions of pain and anxiety but did, in fact, feel better with the help received. Alternatively, there may have been no actual improvement in pain or anxiety but rather a report bias in the direction of pleasing the investigator (especially if the therapists obtained the children's self-reports).

These questions do not have simple answers, but must be considered in any clinical situation or study of children's pain and anxiety. A final question is an ethical one. If children's symptoms are assessed for the investigator's interests (e.g., for an assessment study to "validate" instruments), could questioning children about their pain or anxiety make these symptoms worse? Is it ethical to remind children about their pain if they are coping effectively by not thinking about it or by using distraction?

Our recommendation is to learn from the children in our practice and in our studies. If we ask them, we will find out if our assessments are disruptive and we will learn whether our interventions are beneficial. The most informative measure may not be the numerical quantitative data obtained but the qualitative responses to questions such as: "What bothered you the most?" "What helped you to feel better?" "How did it help you?" etc. Through such questions the quantitative data will gain meaning.

CHEMOTHERAPY-RELATED NAUSEA AND VOMITING

While improvements made in chemotherapeutic agents have increased survival for many children with cancer, problems of nausea and vomiting affect the quality of life and are a major reason for noncompliance leading to treatment failures (Smith, Rosen, Trueworthy, & Lowman, 1979; Zeltzer et al., 1980). Because of these problems and because of the inconsistent and often disappointing effects of antiemetic pharmacologic agents in treating these symptoms, a variety of behavioral interventions for reducing nausea and vomiting have been studied. The majority of these investigations have been conducted in adults with cancer; they have primarily focused on *anticipatory* nausea and vomiting (Redd & Andrykowski, 1982). Assessment methods used in these studies of adults have included self-rating scales of nausea and vomiting, home diaries in which each episode of emesis is recorded, and nurse observation of symptoms.

There have been fewer studies in children receiving chemotherapy. Based on interviews of 80 pediatric patients undergoing chemotherapy, Dolgin et al. (1985) found a 29% prevalence rate for anticipatory nausea and a 20% rate for anticipatory emesis. A significant factor associated with these anticipatory symptoms was the severity of post-chemotherapy nausea and vomiting, a finding similar to that seen in studies of anticipatory nausea and vomiting in adults (Morrow, 1982). In another study, 49 pediatric oncology patients, ages 5 to 21 years, prospectively rated on a 1–10 Likert scale their nausea and vomiting within 3 to 5 days after the administration of each course of chemotherapy (Zeltzer et al., 1984). The extent of emesis in children was not influenced by the number of drugs in the chemotherapeutic regimen. Children's pattern of symptoms did not remain stable during repeated courses of the same agents. There was also wide variation in severity of symptoms among children receiving the same agents. The authors concluded that factors other than the drugs themselves exert a significant influence on chemotherapy-associated nausea and vomiting in children.

Several studies have assessed the efficacy of intervention for these children. In a study of metoclopromide toxicity in hospitalized children receiving chemotherapy, Allen, Gralla, Reilly, Kellick, and Young (1985) also assessed the efficacy of this antiemetic in reducing children's emesis. Nurses recorded children's vomiting episodes, empirically defined as expulsion of vomitus or a timed period of retching. Antiemetic efficacy was classified into four categories, based on a defined number of vomiting episodes. Interestingly, the antiemetic was found to be effective (i.e., less than 5 vomiting episodes) in 70% of newly treated patients, but ineffective in more than 50% of children who had previous experience with chemotherapy.

In a small study of behavioral intervention for adolescents with cancer (Zeltzer, Kellerman, Ellenberg, & Dash, 1983), the assessment instrument was a diary in which adolescents recorded the frequency, severity and duration of their vomiting. The intervention appeared to be effective, based on the diaries returned. However, a subject selection bias was introduced because only a subsample of adolescents accurately completed their diaries. The home diary method was subsequently abandoned in favor of a global rating scale to assess nausea and vomiting. In another pilot study (LeBaron & Zeltzer, 1984a), ratings of nausea and vomiting were obtained from children and their parents by telephone interview within 3 to 5 days after the completion of chemotherapy.

In a comparison study of two behavioral intervention strategies for nausea and vomiting (Zeltzer, LeBaron, & Zeltzer, 1984a), two matched baseline courses of chemotherapy were assessed for 51 children 6 to 17 years of age. The children and their parents each rated (0–10 Likert scale) the severity of nausea and vomiting, and the extent to which chemotherapy "bothered" the child. Data were collected through a telephone interview within 24 hours following the cessation of chemotherapy-related symptoms. The study design called for the assessment of two baseline courses and two with intervention. Assessment of a follow-up course with no intervention was possible for half the patients. While 51 children were enrolled in the study, only 19 patients received intervention. The reason for the relatively small percentage of participants was related to a common methodological problem in intervention studies of children receiving chemotherapy. That is, almost a third (16 patients) were found to have minimal symptoms during baseline assessment and thus did not need intervention. Another 16 patients had their chemotherapy agents or doses altered during the period of the study because of disease relapse or bone marrow toxicity. For studies of intervention in this population, probably three times as many children need to be assessed as deemed necessary for sufficient power, if methodologic rigor is to be maintained in terms of matched courses of chemotherapy. However, while there was the potential for a subject selection bias, the above study did improve upon previous pediatric studies from a methodologic standpoint. Both a comparison group and an internal control (i.e., multiple baseline design) were used, and multiple assessments were made prior to and during intervention. Also, assessment of symptoms was made following termination of intervention to assess endurance of the effects.

Another group of investigators (Cotanch, Hockenberry, & Herman, 1985) compared behavioral intervention to "standard procedure" in 12 adolescents (6 in each group) receiving chemotherapy as inpatients. Two courses of each patient's chemotherapy were assessed using the following measures: (1) vomiting frequency and volume measured by nurses (no mention is made of oral intake prior to chemotherapy); (2) intensity of nausea and vomiting (children's ratings); (3) severity of nausea, and (4) oral intake for 24 hours after drug infusion. The authors reported measuring nausea and vomiting using a thermometer visual analog scale. However, they did not describe or reference this scale. They also differentiated between intensity and severity of nausea, referring to the latter as "the unpleasantness" of the side effect. To obtain a severity score, they used a modification (not described) of a Pain Perception Profile to "psychophysically scale the perception of nausea." They reported that they had to eliminate more than half the scales because the children could not understand them.

Redd, Jacobsen, and Die-Trill (submitted) used videogames during two 10-minute intervals as a distraction intervention for 20 children (9–20 years) with cancer. Measures included a 10 cm visual analog scale for self-ratings of nausea and anxiety. None of the children were reported to have experienced anticipatory emesis. Pulse and blood pressure were also assessed. Intervention occurred for 10 minutes, with another 10 minutes of no intervention, followed by 10 minutes of intervention. Some of the children subsequently received a similar trial at another visit. Nausea and anxiety ratings moved in the expected directions (i.e., lower with intervention) for the first trial but not for the second. Pulse did not change. Systolic blood pressure rose with intervention during the first trial, and diastolic blood pressure significantly decreased when intervention was removed during the second trial. However, the degree of change for both was not clinically significant. This study illustrates again the problems of interpreting physiological data. Presumably the pulse and blood pressure relate to physiological arousal and, if so, they should correlate with level of anxiety and/or discomfort. Since the fluctuations in children's heart rate and blood pressure throughout any clinic visit are unknown, it is very difficult to know how to interpret most physiological data of this sort.

What are the methodological considerations in assessing nausea and vomiting? The first consideration is to distinguish anticipatory symptoms from those which occur following the administration of chemotherapy. Studies in adults focus assessment and intervention on the former, since these symptoms occur for the most part in the clinic setting and are thus presumably easier to assess. On the other hand, the few studies in children have focused primarily on the latter (i.e., post-chemotherapy side effects). Assessment methods may differ according to which of the above symptoms are studied.

Anticipatory nausea and vomiting are believed to be conditioned responses usually associated with past experiences of severe post-chemotherapy nausea and vomiting (Andrykowski, Redd, & Hartfield, 1985; Dolgin, Katz, McGinty, & Siegel, 1985; Morrow, 1982). Patients' level of anxiety is assumed to play a role in adults (Morrow, 1982; VanKomen & Redd, 1985), but this association has not yet been adequately assessed in children. Children's level of anxiety moved in the same direction as nausea in the study by Redd et al. (submitted), but numerical values were much lower for anxiety than for nausea. These data are difficult to interpret since the gradations and endpoints of the visual analog scales used were not reported. If anxiety is found to be an important contributor to anticipatory nausea and vomiting in children, then the technical difficulty encountered in administering the chemotherapy needs to be noted. For example, for most children a needle inserted in the vein successfully during the first "stick" is easier to cope with than a series of unsuccessful sticks. Another factor relating to drug administration is the form of the administration (i.e., intravenous push versus slow drip). For example, some drugs which are given by intravenous push are associated with certain cues not found when drugs are given over several hours by slow drip method. Such cues include a specific taste in the mouth and a burning sensation along the vein (especially when the drug is pushed rapidly). Not uncommonly, we have seen children begin vomiting as an *antiemetic* was being pushed intravenously, before any chemotherapy had been given. When questioned later, the children had assumed that the antiemetic was one of the chemotherapy drugs. Another visual cue is the color of the drug. For children with anticipatory nausea and vomiting with doxorubicin (red color), for example, the response to changes such as covering the medication bottles or even coloring the antiemetic red would help determine the extent to which drug color is a significant visual cue for those children. These and other chemotherapy administration factors need to be taken into account when studying anticipatory symptoms. In studies of intervention, such cues for anticipatory symptoms need to be indentified and controlled as best as possible so that they do not confound the findings related to efficacy of the intervention.

The next consideration is how to *assess* nausea and vomiting. For anticipatory emesis and post-chemotherapy emesis in hospitalized children, a seemingly simple solution might be to observe and count emeses. These data are not as objective as they may appear. First, there are individual differences in the definition of a "vomit." In their study of an antiemetic, Allen et al. (1985) defined vomit as "explusion of any vomitus or up to five nonproductive retches within a five-minute period." Yet some children accumulate enough saliva in their mouth to have this be confused with gastric contents (although fastidious investigators could assess the pH of the material to differentiate the two). Also, retching (also known as "dry heaves") may occur when the stomach is empty. Should retching then be considered different from vomiting from a clinical distress standpoint? Although some investigators have measured volume of vomitus in an attempt to be objective, they have not considered the patient's oral intake. This important variable affects gastric content. For children who intermittently retch and vomit, the observed and recorded emesis count may be influenced by the severity of the child's distress while vomiting. That is, we have found that an observer is likely to record a higher number of emeses for a child who vomits with much distress than for the child who is less bothered by the same amount of vomiting.

Assessment of post-chemotherapy emesis for children who receive their chemotherapy as outpatients presents another logistical problem, since these children may vomit in the car and at home for several hours to several days. Parents are not "independent" observers, and constant monitoring of their children for the purpose of data collection may not be advisable. When self-recording of adolescents' symptoms was attempted by use of a structured home diary (Zeltzer et al., 1983), only a subsample returned completed (and trustworthy) diaries. Some reported that they "forgot their diaries" or were seen to be completing them retrospectively in the clinic waiting room. Also, whether parent or child is responsible for maintaining the diary, a daily focus on nausea and vomiting for the sake of recording each noxious event is the antithesis of most intervention strategies. Interventions generally encourage a focus of attention *away* from feelings of discomfort. Yet, somehow these symptoms must be assessed if effects of intervention are to be evaluated. Furthermore, *nausea* cannot be observed in either the hospital or at home. The child must be relied upon to report the occurrence and severity of this event.

For all of these reasons, parent and child ratings of nausea and vomiting are obtained in our studies through structured telephone interviews following the last day of post-chemotherapy nausea and vomiting. We have found that parents and their children agree at least 80% of the time (Zeltzer et al., 1984a) in their ratings of the child's nausea and vomiting. It seems as if children's ratings are not totally idiosyncratic. However, developmental abilities must be considered in assessing the validity of children's ratings. That is, at what age can children understand and use a rating scale to describe the extent and duration of their nausea and vomiting? Not only are children called upon to translate experience into a series of numbers which each have a different abstract meaning to the investigator, but their concept of time and their short-term memory for unpleasant symptoms also come into play. Additionally, how does the extent of suffering influence the child's use of a rating scale for nausea and vomiting? When we administered a series of nausea/vomiting vignettes to healthy school children, we found that even first graders were able to differentiate a small amount of nausea and vomiting from a large amount occurring over a longer period of time (Zeltzer, LeBaron, & Richie, submitted). The accuracy with which children were able to fine tune their ratings increased with increasing age from first through fifth grade. Thus, it appears that healthy children in a non-medical environment can understand and utilize a rating scale for symptoms such as nausea and vomiting. This study needs to be replicated in children who are receiving chemotherapy to determine the extent to which children's personal experience with nausea and vomiting influences their ratings.

It is obviously important not only to quantify nausea and vomiting, but also to assess functional outcomes, such as the extent of disruption of eating, play, school, and sleep. The issue of the extent to which nausea and vomiting bothers children is an important one. Some children may vomit ten times and have their day totally disrupted. Others will vomit a similar number of times and yet be able to continue with normal activities. "Suffering" (bother) and functional (i.e., school, play, sleep, etc.) components of the assessment should be included in studies of intervention for children receiving chemotherapy.

CONCLUSION

Assessment of children's pain, anxiety, nausea, and vomiting has some special features which differentiate it from similar information gathering in adults. Developmental differences relating to cognitive abilities and life experience influence what can be asked of the child and how the child's behaviors are to be interpreted. As children get older, they display their suffering in a more goal-directed manner and with more behavioral control. Thus, self-reports become essential, especially in the assessment of pain. Nausea and vomiting may be even more difficult to assess. Dichotomization of vomiting as "objective" data and nausea as "subjective" data can lead the investigator down a path of biased or uninterpretable findings. The best way to assess nausea and vomiting in children is yet to be determined. However, it is clear that purely physical quantification of nausea and vomiting does not tell the whole story (or perhaps even the most important story). Data regarding the amount of suffering related to these symptoms and the extent to which they disrupt the child's daily life may be far more meaningful for most patients.

Decisions about the use of observational, physiological, and self-assessment methods for any of the above symptoms must be based on the clinical and research questions asked. Too often, findings are statistically significant but their clinical meaning is uninterpretable within the context of the study. In the search for "hard data" in what is frequently called a "soft science," behavioral scientists often forget the value of gathering descriptive data. Such information is invaluable in helping to interpret the objective data. A balance between qualitative and quantitative data is what makes a study rich and meaningful.

REFERENCES

Abu-Saad, H. & Holzemer, W. L. (1981). Measuring children's self-assessment of pain. *Issues in Comprehensive Pediatric Nursing, 5,* 337–349.
Allen, J. C., Gralla, R., Reilly, L., Kellick, M., & Young, C. (1985). Metoclopramide: Dose-related toxicity and preliminary antiemetic studies in children receiving cancer chemotherapy. *Journal of Clinical Oncology, 3,* 1136–1141.

Andrykowski, M. A., Redd, W. H., & Hartfield, A. K. (1985). Development of anticipatory nausea: A prospective analysis. *Journal of Consulting and Clinical Psychology, 53,* 447–454.

Cotanch, P., Hockenberry, M., & Herman, S. (1985). Self-Hypnosis as antiemetic therapy in children receiving chemotherapy. *Oncology Nursing Forum, 12,* 41–46.

Craig, K. D., McMahon, R. J., Morison, J. D., & Zaskow, C. (1984). Developmental changes in infant pain expression during immunization injections. *Social Science and Medicine, 19,* 1331–1337.

Dolgin, M. J., Katz, E. R., McGinty, K., & Siegel, S. E. (1985). Anticipatory nausea and vomiting in pediatric cancer patients. *Pediatrics, 75,* 547–552.

Eland, J. M. (1981). Minimizing pain associated with prekindergarten intramuscular injections. *Issues in Comprehensive Pediatric Nursing, 5,* 361–372.

Eland, J. M. & Anderson, J. E. (1977). The experience of pain in children. In A. K. Jacox (Ed.), *Pain: A source book for nurses and other health professionals* (pp. 453–473). Boston: Little, Brown and Company.

Harpin, V. A. & Rutter, N. (1982). Development of emotional sweating in the newborn infant. *Archives of Disease in Childhood, 57,* 691–695.

Hilgard, J. R. & LeBaron, S. (1984). *Hypnotherapy of pain in children with Cancer.* Los Altos, California: William Kaufmann, Inc.

Hilgard, J. R. & LeBaron, S. (1982). Relief of anxiety and pain in children and adolescents with cancer: Quantitative measures and clinical observations. *International Journal of Clinical and Experimental Hypnosis, 30,* 417–442.

Jay, S. M. & Elliott, C. (1984). Behavioral observation scales for measuring children's distress: The effects of increased methodological rigor. *Journal of Consulting and Clinical Psychology, 52,* 1106–1107.

Jay, S. M. & Elliott, C. (1986). Multimodal assessment of children's distress during painful medical procedures. Poster session at Society of Behavioral Medicine, San Francisco.

Jay, S., Elliott, C., Katz, E., & Siegel, S. (1985). Distress in children undergoing painful medical procedures: Results of a treatment outcome study. In J. W. Varni (Chair), Comprehensive assessment and management of acute and chronic pain in children. Presented at the Association for the Advancement of Behavioral Therapy, Houston.

Jay, S. M., Ozolins, M., Elliott, C. H., & Caldwell, S. (1983). Assessment of children's distress during painful medical procedures. *Health Psychology, 2,* 133–147.

Jeans, M. E. (1983). Pain in children—a neglected area. In P. Firestone, P. J. McGrath, and W. Feldman (Eds.), *Advances in behavioral medicine for children and adolescents* (pp. 23–37). Hillsdale, New Jersey: Lawrence Erlbaum Associates.

Katz, E. R., Kellerman, J., & Ellenberg, L. (submitted). Hypnosis in the reduction of acute pain and distress in children with cancer undergoing aversive medical procedures.

Katz, E. R., Kellerman, J., & Siegel, S. E. (1980). Behavioral distress in children with cancer undergoing medical procedures: Developmental considerations. *Journal of Consulting and Clinical Psychology, 48,* 356–365.

Katz, E. R., Kellerman, J., & Siegel, S. E. (1981). Anxiety as an effective focus in the clinical study of acute behavioral distress: A reply to Sacham and Daut. *Journal of Consulting and Clinical Psychology, 49,* 470–471.

Katz, E. R., Varni, J. W., & Jay, S. M. (1984). Behavioral assessment and management of pediatric pain. *Progress in Behavioral Modification, 18,* 163–193.

Kellerman, J., Zeltzer, L., Ellenberg, L., & Dash, J. (1983). Adolescents with cancer: Hypnosis for the reduction of the acute pain and anxiety associated with medical procedures. *Journal of Adolescent Health Care, 4,* 85–90.

LeBaron, S. & Zeltzer, L. (1984). Assessment of acute pain and anxiety in children and adolescents by self-reports, observer reports, and a behavior checklist. *Journal of Consulting and Clinical Psychology, 52,* 729–738.

LeBaron, S. & Zeltzer, L. (1984a). Behavioral intervention for reducing chemotherapy-related nausea and vomiting in adolescents with cancer. *Journal of Adolescent Health Care, 5,* 178–182.

Levine, J. D. & Gordon, N. C. (1982). Pain in prelingual children and its evaluation by pain-induced vocalization. *Pain, 14,* 85–93.

Lollar, D. J., Smits, S. J., & Patterson, D. L. (1982). Assessment of pediatric pain: An empirical perspective. *Journal of Pediatric Psychology, 7,* 267–277.

Morrow, G. R. (1982). Prevalence and correlates of anticipatory nausea and vomiting in chemotherapy patients. *Journal of the National Cancer Institute, 68,* 585–588.

Redd, W. H. & Andrykowski, M. A. (1982). Behavioral intervention in cancer treatment: Controlling aversion reactions to chemotherapy. *Journal of Consulting and Clinical Psychology, 50,* 1018–1029.

Redd, W. H., Jacobsen, P. B., & Die-Trill, M. (submitted). Cognitive/Attentional distraction in the control of conditioned nausea in pediatric cancer patients receiving chemotherapy.

Ross, D. M. & Ross, S.A. (1984). The importance of type of question, psychological climate and subject set in interviewing children about pain. *Pain, 19,* 71–79.

Ross, D. M. & Ross, S. A. (1984a). Childhood pain: The school-aged child's viewpoint. *Pain, 20,* 179–191.

Sacham, S. & Daut, R. (1981). Anxiety or pain: What does the scale measure? *Journal of Consulting and Clinical Psychology, 49,* 468–469.

Schultz, N. V. (1971). How children perceive pain. *Nursing Outlook, 19,* 670–673.

Smith, S. D., Rosen, D., Trueworthy, R. C., & Lowman, J. T. (1979). A reliable method for evaluating drug compliance in children with cancer. *Cancer, 43,* 169–173.

VanKomen, R.W. & Redd, W.H. (1985). Personality factors associated with anticipatory nausea/vomiting in patients receiving cancer chemotherapy. *Health Psychology, 4,* 189–202.

Wasz-Hockert, O., Lind, J., Vuorenkoski, V., Partanen, T., & Valanne, E. (1968). The infant cry. In *Clinics in developmental medicine,* No. 29. London: Heinemann; Philadelphia: Lippincott.

White, I. B. & Stow, P. (1985). Rationale and experience with visual analogue toys. *Anaesthesia, 40,* 601–603.

Winer, G. A. (1982). A review and analysis of children's fearful behavior in dental settings. *Child Development, 53,* 1111–1133.

Wolff, P. H. (1969). The natural history of crying and other vocalizations in infancy. In B. M. Foss (Ed.), *Determinants of Infant Behavior* (Vol. 4) (pp. 81–109). London: Methuen.

Zeltzer, L., Kellerman, J., Ellenberg, L., & Dash, J. (1983). Hypnosis for reduction of vomiting associated with chemotherapy and disease in adolescents with cancer. *Journal of Adolescent Health Care, 4,* 77–84.

Zeltzer, L., Kellerman, J., Ellenberg, L., Dash, J., & Rigler, D. (1980). Psychological effects of illness in adolescence. II. Impact of illness in adolescents—crucial issues and coping styles. *Journal of Pediatrics, 97,* 132–138.

Zeltzer, L. & LeBaron, S. (1982). Hypnosis and nonhypnotic techniques for reduction of pain and anxiety during painful procedures in children and adolescents with cancer. *Journal of Pediatrics, 101,* 1032–1035.

Zeltzer, L., LeBaron, S., & Richie, M. (submitted). Validity of self-assessment of nausea and vomiting in children.

Zeltzer, L., LeBaron, S., & Zeltzer, P. M. (1984). A prospective assessment of chemotherapy-related nausea and vomiting in children with cancer. *American Journal of Pediatric Hematology/Oncology, 6,* 5–16.

Zeltzer, L., LeBaron, S., & Zeltzer, P. M. (1984a). The effectiveness of behavioral intervention for reduction of nausea and vomiting in children and adolescents receiving chemotherapy. *Journal of Clinical Oncology, 2,* 683–690.

Zeskind, P. S., Sale, J., Maio, M. L., Huntington, L., & Weiseman, J. R. (1985). Adult perceptions of pain and hunger cries: A synchrony of arousal. *Child Development, 56,* 549–554.

Assessment of Cognitive Function in Cancer Patients

Thomas E. Oxman
Paula P. Schnurr
Peter M. Silberfarb

ABSTRACT. Cognitive function comprises the brain's integrative powers to acquire, process, store, and retrieve information. Normal cognitive function is necessary for the cancer patient to relate history accurately, comprehend and follow treatment recommendations, and give informed consent for diagnostic, therapeutic, and research purposes. Deficits in cognitive function imply the presence of an organic mental syndrome that is the result of abnormalities in cerebral physiology or structure. Because some of the etiologic factors of organic mental syndromes can be reduced or eliminated, those caring for cancer patients should be alert for cognitive impairment in its earliest stages. In this article, we will critically review methods currently in use for assessing cognitive function, emphasizing those most relevant for cancer patients.

INTRODUCTION

Cognitive function comprises the brain's integrative power to acquire, process, store, and retrieve information. Cognitive function thus includes awareness, attention, memory, perception, orientation, comprehension, and abstraction. Deficits in cognitive function imply the presence of an organic mental syndrome that is the result of abnormalities in cerebral physiology or structure (Folstein, Fetting, Lobo, Unaiza & Capozzoli, 1984; Lipowski, 1980; Silberfarb, 1983).

Normal cognitive function is necessary to allow an individual to manage daily activities. It is particularly important for

Thomas E. Oxman, MD, Paula P. Schnurr, PhD, and Peter M. Silberfarb, MD may be contacted at the Department of Psychiatry, Dartmouth Medical School, Hanover, NH 03756.

the cancer patient so that he or she can relate history accurately, comprehend and follow treatment recommendations, and give informed consent for diagnostic, therapeutic, and research procedures.

Cognitive deficits are common in cancer patients who have experienced metastases to the central nervous system (Silberfarb, 1983). However, primary central nervous system tumors or cerebral metastases from other sites need not be present in order for deficits in cognition to occur. In general, the etiology of cognitive impairment is usually multifactorial; medications, fever, infection, side effects of therapy, nutritional deficiencies, and metabolic and endocrinological abnormalities all pose threats to the central nervous system. Also, because cancer patients are living longer than they did in the past (Fries, 1980; Silberfarb, 1983), some are likely to reach an age at which they are susceptible to cognitive impairment if challenged by any of the aforementioned stresses. The fact that some of these etiologic factors of organic mental syndromes can be reduced or eliminated is the crucial reason why those caring for cancer patients should be alert for cognitive impairment in its earliest stages. In this article we will critically review methods currently in use for assessing cognitive function, emphasizing those that are most applicable with cancer patients.

ORGANIC MENTAL SYNDROMES

Organic mental syndromes are a cluster of psychological and behavioral symptoms caused by destruction of cerebral neurons and of their transient metabolic dysfunction (Lipowski, 1978). Delirium and dementia are the most common of these syndromes. The primary symptoms of delirium amd dementia involve global information processing and result in or are accompanied by emotional and motivational disturbances. Occasionally, the emotional and motivational problems are the only symptoms. Physicians and nurses sometimes focus on these other behaviors and erroneously attribute them to a patient's reaction to the meaning of cancer (Goodwin, Goodwin & Kellner, 1979; Levine, Silberfarb & Lipowski, 1978). Although the topic is relatively neglected, the prevalence of organic mental disorders in cancer patients ranges from 28 to 79 percent in terminal patients and 40 percent of consecutive patients referred for psychiatric consultation (Lipowski, 1980).

Delirium is a transient and fluctuating mental disorder reflecting acute brain failure due to widespread derangement of cerebral metabolism (Lipowski, 1980). It is one of the most frequently encountered organic mental syndromes in the general population (McEvoy, 1981). Although the onset is sudden and the duration averages one week, delirium may be followed by coma and death (Lipowski, 1978; Rabins & Folstein, 1982; Whybrow & Spencer, 1969). Due to this association with mortality, it is important to search for early, subtle changes in behavior in order to allow early diagnosis and treatment.

The diagnostic criteria for delirium incorporated in DSM-III (American Psychiatric Association, 1980) are the following:

1. Clouding of consciousness, defined as reduced clarity of awareness of the environment associated with reduced capacity to shift, focus and sustain attention;
2. At least 2 of following: perceptual disturbance, speech that is incoherent at times, disturbance of sleep-wakefulness cycle, increased or decreased psychomotor activity;
3. Disorientation and memory impairment, if testable;
4. Clinical features that develop over hours to days and fluctuate;
5. Evidence from history, physical, or laboratory tests of a specific factor judged etiological.

Delirium is one of the potential remote manifestations of a neoplasm outside the brain. Treatment modalities, such as narcotics or chemotherapy, can also cause delirium. Not surprisingly, within a group of cancer patients suffering organic mental syndromes, Levine et al. (1978) diagnosed 20% as probably having CNS metastases as the cause and 80% as having a metabolic or toxic disturbance as the cause.

Dementia usually is an insidious, destructive process with higher cortical dysfunction as the most prominent symptom. Changes in arousal and attention are relatively terminal features. Although clear separation of delirium and dementia is to some extent arbitrary, the diagnostic criteria for dementia in DSM-III include:

1. A loss of intellectual abilities of sufficient severity to interfere with social or occupational functioning;
2. Memory impairment;
3. At least one of the following: (a) impairment of abstract thinking (b) impaired judgement (c) other disturbances of higher cortical function such as aphasia and apraxia;
4. State of consciousness that is not clouded as in delirium or intoxication, although these may be superimposed.

Patients with cerebral tumors commonly present with symptoms of raised intracranial pressure, focal neurological signs, or seizures, all of which are likely to result in direct evaluation by a neurologist or neurosurgeon. Nevertheless, primary central nervous system tumors can result in a subtle presentation of dementia. Lishman (1978) has concluded that slow growing central nervous system tumors tend to allow premorbid personality traits to exaggerate while patients with faster growing tumors present with more global cognitive defects in the form of a mild dementia. Furthermore, long-term cognitive effects of some chemotherapeutic agents (e.g., intrathecal methotrexate as used to treat acute leukemias) have also recently been reported as dementia in previously treated childhood leukemics (Meadows & Evans, 1976).

METHODS OF ASSESSMENT

Clinical History and Observation

Adequate historical information about the cancer patient's past life and premorbid personality is the cornerstone for all other methods of cognitive assessment. For example, answers to mental status questions or questionnaires must be interpreted in light of a person's occupation and education. Moreover, premorbid personality traits are often amplified by delirium and mold its expression.

Careful observation of a patient's verbal and nonverbal behavior and sleep are important to make on a daily basis.

Subtle changes, if interpreted in the context of his or her premorbid personality and behavior, can provide the first indications of a developing delirium. For example, difficulty finding the correct word when talking, slight forgetfulness, misidentification of persons or surroundings, and complaints of difficulty concentrating are important verbal cues of delirium. The observation of abnormal psychomotor behavior, ranging from the extreme of purposeless hyperactivity to catatonic stupor with abrupt shifts to either side of the spectrum, can also facilitate the diagnosis of an organic mental syndrome. Alteration of the normal sleep-waking cycle is another clue, often overlooked. Insomnia is the most common alteration, but reversal of the cycle is also probable with drowsiness during daytime and insomnia at night. Emotional behaviors, such as a reduced ability to cope with new or complex tasks, anxiety or anger in common social situations, and socially inappropriate acts, are also clues to a potential organic mental syndrome.

The Formal Bedside Mental Status Examination

The mental status examination is part of a complete medical history and physical examination. It depends upon the description and evaluation of observable behavioral responses. One of its most important purposes is to provide an accurate description of a patient's current mental functioning. This description is an important baseline for later comparisons. The mental status examination includes tests of cognitive functioning as well as the description of the patient's appearance, general behavior, motor activity, speech, alertness, mood, the views he or she holds about his or her condition, the attitude displayed throughout the examination, the reactions evoked by the patient in the examiner, and observations regarding the patient's behavior toward members of his family and medical personnel.

The cognitive portion of the mental status examination consists largely of test questions from different psychometric tests. For detection of organic mental sydromes, the most important aspects that can be readily tested are orientation, attention and concentration, memory, and abstraction. Some common questions used to test those cognitive functions are outlined in Appendix A (Keller & Manschreck, 1981; Matarazzo, 1972; Melges, 1975; Strub & Black, 1977). Three general principles apply to asking all of these questions. First, the examiner should make the patient feel as comfortable as possible; the cancer patient should be told that this is a routine part of the history and physical examination in order to periodically assess for possible effects of drugs or tumors on his or her concentration and memory. Second, easy questions in a series should be asked before harder ones; also, encouragement by the examiner is appropriate. Third, except for orientation, a patient should not be given the correct answers to questions he or she has failed in order to decrease effects on repeated testing.

Brief Standardized Cognitive Screening Examinations

Uniformity and reliability of data, along with a reduction of examiner bias, are obvious advantages to using a structured cognitive examination for research purposes. If a structured cognitive examination could be made brief and easy to administer, then it could also provide a means for increasing the low frequency of routine clinical checking of cognitive function (Helzer, 1981; Jacobs, Bernhard, Delgado & Strain, 1977). Accordingly, increased efforts are being made to develop and evaluate such instruments.

Standardized cognitive examinations range from an extensive three hour neuropsychological battery (Rietan & Davison, 1974) to a 5 minute questionnaire (Kahn, Goldfarb, Pollack & Peck, 1960). Because of the need to screen large numbers of patients and the decreased concentrating capacity of delirious patients, more attention has been appropriately given to the use of briefer questionnaires as screening instruments for further cognitive and neurological evaluation. Appendix B lists several of these briefer screens, a selection of which are discussed below.

The Mini-Mental State Exam

The Mini-Mental State Examination was developed by Folstein, Folstein and McHugh (1975) as a practical method for the clinician to grade the cognitive state of patients. It is used to assess a subject's orientation, recall, short-term memory, and concentration. Unlike several other similar cognitive screening tests, it also includes questions of higher level nonverbal as well as verbal cognitive functions. The items contained in the examination are shown in Appendix C. A score is derived from summing the points for each completed task, so that potential scores range from 0-30. This exam may be administered by clinical or lay personnel with little training. It usually requires less than five minutes for completion. The examiner (psychiatric resident, nurse, volunteer, etc.) is instructed to make the patient comfortable, establish rapport, praise successes, and avoid pressing on items which the patient has difficulty answering correctly. The exam is divided into two sections. In the first part, which has a maximum score of 21, the patient must provide vocal responses. The second part, which has a maximum score of 9, tests ability to name, follow commands, write, and copy a figure. A total score of 20 or less is usually found only in dementia, delirium, schizophrenia or affective disorder.

The Cognitive Capacity Screening Examination

Jacobs et al. (1977) developed a similar brief examination for testing medical patients. Like the Mini-Mental Status Exam, it was designed to take approximately five minutes for completion. Unlike the Mini-Mental Status Exam, it was designed more specifically to detect delirium. Because a global impairment such as delirium should influence the patient's ability to shift tasks, the order in which questions are presented is designed to require rapid shifts from one task to another. The 30 items of the questionnaire are shown in Appendix D. As with the Mini-Mental State Exam, the cutoff point for cognitive impairment is 20.

Neuropsychological Testing

Some parts of the bedside mental status examination (for example, digit span) are subtests of longer neuropsychological tests. Extensive psychometric testing, such as Reitan's modification of the Halstead Battery (Reitan & Davison, 1974), provides a fairly precise estimate of cognitive function. The length and cost of standardized neuropsychological testing, however,

preclude its use in routine screening examination. Nevertheless, subtests of neuropsychological batteries are often recommended for improved quantification of cognitive function and
for monitoring changes in organic mental impairment.

One good example of such a test is the Trail Making Test
(Conn, 1977; Oxman & Silberfarb, 1980). A conventional
Trail Making Test has two parts. In the first part, a subject is
given a sheet of paper on which there are 25 consecutively
numbered circles from 1 to 25 and told to connect the circles
in order as quickly as possible; practice on a series of 8 is
given prior to the administration of the test. The time to
complete the full series is taken as the score, with a score
from 13 to 75 seconds considered normal. In the second part,
which is more difficult, there are 13 numbered circles and 12
circles with letters A to L. The subject must alternate between numbers and letters in ascending sequence (1,A,2,B,
3,C . . .) as quickly as possible (normal time = 19-180 secs).
In both versions, errors must be corrected and are thus incorporated in the time score. Normal scores vary somewhat with
age, so age-graded norms should be used for the interpretation of a given patient's score (Lezak, 1976). Performance on
the test is likely to be affected by brain disorders in many
different locations because the test requires spatial analysis,
motor control, ability to shift attention, alertness, concentration, and number and letter sense.

Three other related examples are the Bender Visual Motor Gestalt Test (Bender, 1938), the Benton Visual Retention Test (Benton, 1963), and the Graham Kendall Memory
for Designs Test (Graham & Kendall, 1960). In the Bender-
Gestalt Test, nine simple designs are presented on cards for
the patient to copy, one at a time. The type and frequency
of errors are noted, The Benton Visual Retention Test differs primarily in that the subject must draw a geometric
design from memory after having seen the design on a card
for a given length of time. The test thus requires short-term
retention and recall, as well as spatio-constructive abilities. It
can be made more difficult by using shorter card exposures.
Performance is scored by the number of cards correctly re-
produced and by the number of errors. Graham and Kendall's test is similar but allows for tranforming raw scores
into scores which control for the effects of age and IQ.

Neurological Signs

Abnormal neurological physical signs are frequently seen in patients with cognitive deficits. Over 30 inter-related neurological signs have been associated with diffuse cognitive impairment, usually of a more chronic duration such as in dementia. These signs are primarily either primitive reflexes (Basavaraju, Silverstone, Libow & Paraskevas, 1981; Jenkyn, Walsh, Culver, & Reeves, 1977; Kaufman, Wienberger, Strain & Jacobs, 1979) or abnormal perceptual-sensory responses (Bender, 1975; Brink, Bryant, Catalano, Janakes & Oliveira, 1979; Fink, Green & Bender, 1952; Kurucz, Feldmar & Werner, 1979). Many of these signs are normally present during early central nervous system maturation and reappear with age or diffuse cerebral disease.

The face-hand test (Fink et al., 1952), also known as double simultaneous stimulation, requires the patient to close his or her eyes and describe where he or she is touched by the examiner. The examiner alternately touches the cheek, then the cheek and dorsum of the hand simultaneously. Ten trials are given with 8 face-hand combinations of 4 contralateral and 4 ipsilateral stimuli, and 2 interspersed combinations of hand-hand and face-face. If a patient fails consistently to locate both stimuli correctly, the response is considered abnormal. The main types of errors are improper localization or extinguishing of one of the places stimulated.

Basavaraju et al. (1981) and Jenkyn et al. (1977) have investigated brief screening batteries of these neurological signs for use during the physical examination. The more discriminating of the primitive reflexes are shown in Appendix E. Testing of these reflexes may be easily incorporated into the physical examination with minimal expenditure of time.

EVALUATION OF METHODS

The examiner is a major source of variation in performance on all of the tests reviewed above. Observational skill should, however, improve with training and practice (Kaplan, 1984). Depending on the particular discipline of the examiner and the types of cancer patients in a particular setting, the examiner should be able to establish an appropriate routine of cognitive evaluation from among the different methods. In order to select appropriate tests, it is important to be aware of the limitations of each method.

Mental Status Examination

Despite having been developed over 80 years ago, tests such as serial sevens, memory tests, and proverb interpretations have not been established as valid assessments of higher intellectual functions. Nevertheless, several reports offer useful guidelines. In their review of the bedside mental status examination, Keller and Manshreck (1981) confirm that orientation is usually lost first to time, then place, and rarely to person. Testing of orientation can be performed with between and within rater reliability. Memory tests are quite reliable but by themselves are not vaild in establishing an organic diagnosis because these tests are strongly dependent on intelligence, age, and mood. However, when (a) premorbid history is well known, (b) other psychiatric disorders are of low probability, and (c) cooperation is adequate, memory tests such as recall of objects at 2 or 5 minutes and memory for remote personal events and recent general events are certainly useful for identifying organic mental syndromes.

High reliability and validity for bedside tests of attention and concentration have yet to be reported. The Serial Sevens Test, for example, was originally designed as a test of intelligence in children; it is currently used as a test of ability to attend to a task (Manning, 1982). Moreover, discriminating norms have been difficult to establish; when the Serial Sevens Test of Kraepelin was given to normals, 58% made errors (Keller & Manschreck, 1981).

Because intelligence has a strong effect on performance on tests of higher intellectual functioning, assessment of intelligence is an important part of the mental status examination. Unfortunately, there are no clinical tests that can be performed in several minutes to permit a precise estimate of intelligence. Useful estimates can be made from inquiring about the patient's performance in school, level of occupational attainment, vocabulary, and ability to manage abstract

ideas. If there are major inconsistencies among these historical features and clinical observations, more formal neuropsychological testing may be indicated. As an intermediary
step, the clinician can use the general information or vocabulary subtests of the WAIS (Melges, 1975; Strub & Black,
1977).

Proverb interpretation is one part of the mental status examination that is often used to identify and discriminate
among thought disorders. Bizarre and idiosyncratic responses
are more characteristic of schizophrenia, clang associations of
mania, and concrete responses of organic brain syndromes.
Unfortunately, the interrater reliability of proverb interpretation tests is low (Andreasen, 1977). Proverbs used in intelligence tests, however, have adequate reliability and validity
(Wechsler, 1972). Reich (1981) demonstrated the value of
giving at least four proverbs to increase interrater reliability
for discriminating hospitalized psychiatric patients and hospitalized nonpsychiatric patients.

As mentioned above, intact judgment is especially important to the cancer patient. The evaluation of judgment is traditionally included in mental status testing by interpreting
responses to hypothetical situations, such as what should you
do if you find an addressed envelope? There is no evidence
that responses to these situations will indicate cognitive impairment without there being grosser disturbances on other
tests (Keller & Manschreck, 1981). Moreover, the relationship between answers to such questions and the types of judg-
ments necessary for the cancer patients' daily or long-term life
goals has not been established. Accordingly, it is better to
inquire about these areas directly and concentrate the formal
mental status questions on those areas that are known to be
more reliable and valid (Keller & Manschreck, 1981).

It appears that the most important finding regarding the
mental status exam is that its components should not be used
in isolation (as is often done by busy house staff who might
only ask questions about orientation). Doing so can greatly
increase false negative findings. For example, Talland (1965)
found that even patients with Korsakoff's psychosis perform
adequately on digit span testing. Such problems have led investigators like Folstein et al. (1975) and Jacobs et al. (1977)
to develop structured mental status examinations.

Brief Standardized Mental Status Examinations

As illustrated in Appendix B, numerous standardized brief mental status examinations are reported in the literature. Most of the more recently developed ones are for more specific use in detecting or following dementia. Of those developed for use in general medical populations, no one is superior to the other on a priori grounds. Some, such as the Mini-Mental State Exam and Taylor, Abrams, Faber and Almy's (1980) battery, were designed theoretically to assess different cortical functional regions. In practice, however, these instruments appear better suited for detecting diffuse cortical dysfunction (Dick, Guloff, Steward, Blackstock, Bielawska, Paul & Marsden, 1984; Tsai & Tsuang, 1979; Webster, Scott, Nunn, McNeer & Varnell, 1984).

Because the Mini-Mental State Exam was selected as part of the lay administered Diagnostic Interview Schedule contracted by the National Institute of Mental Health, it has been given to 15,000 people in five cities as part of the epidemiologic catchment survey program. Ninety-five percent of these individuals scored in the range of 24 to 30. When used in 100 consecutive cases on general medical inpatient unit, a cut-off score of 23 or 24 gives maximum specificity and sensitivity (Folstein et al., 1984). The Mini-Mental State Exam separated three diagnostic groups from each other and a normal group: The mean score was 9.7 for dementia, 19 for depression with cognitive impairment, 25.1 for uncomplicated affective disorder, and 27.6 for normals (Folstein et al., 1975). In a second sample of 137 consecutive admissions, the mean scores were: dementia, 12.2; affective disorder depressed, 25.9; mania, 26.6; schizophrenia, 24.6; personality disorders, 26.8; and neuroses, 27.6. Test scores were reliable on 24 hour and 28 day retest. In a study of 99 consecutively admitted general medical patients, sensitivity for delirium and dementia was 87% while specificity was 82% (Anthony, LeResche, Niaz, von Korff & Folstein, 1982).

Neuropsychological Subtests

Neuropsychological tests vary in the degree to which they have been validated. For specific use in cancer patients there are no adequate norms that have been established. However, because these tests can be given with strict standardization, the possibility of establishing norms for cancer patients is promising. The danger that accompanies this promise is failure to interpret results in light of all other historical and clinical information about the individual cancer patient.

A major disadvantage of the Trail Making test is that results may be affected by poor eyesight or, if present, cumbersome or painful intravenous tubing attached to a patient's writing arm. Nevertheless, Reitan (1958) demonstrated that loss of the skills tested by this instrument, such as the ability to integrate numbers and letters, may be one of the earliest symptoms of delirium. Therefore, poor eyesight or the presence of intravenous tubing should not prevent the clinician from using the Trail Making Test in diagnostic assessment, but these factors should be taken into account, especially in the interpretation of marginally poor scores. A practice effect has been demonstrated when the Trails B was given 20 times over a 10 week period, but depending on how frequently such a test is repeated, it can be used to measure changes in mental status (Conn, 1977; Oxman & Silberfarb, 1980).

As with many of the bedside tests, many of the neuropsychological tests are significantly correlated with intelligence. Nevertheless, among perceptual sensory tests, the Bender-Gestalt Visual-Motor Test, the Graham Kendall Memory for Designs Test, and the Benton Visual Retention test have received support for detection of organic mental syndromes (Brilliant & Gynther, 1963; Eslinger, Damasio, Benton & Van Allen, 1985; Yates, 1966). One of the important issues in evaluating these tests, however, is to know the base rate of organic mental syndrome in the clinical groups of interest. In a comparative study of these three tests for organicity in a psychiatric population, the non-organic base rate was 70% (Brilliant & Gynther, 1963). The accuracy of the Bender and Benton-error scores were 82% and 66% respectively. Therefore, the Bender resulted in a 12% increase over just assuming the base rate, while the Benton-error score, a good diagnostic guideline, led to a decrease in accuracy compared to assuming the base rate.

Neurological Signs

Both Basavaraju et al. (1981) and Jenkyn et al. (1977) have formally tested the value of a battery of primitive reflexes for detection of cerebral dysfunction. Focusing primarily on dementia, Basavaraju et al. found that the face-hand test along with the large-small figure perception test were best able to discriminate between healthy elderly and cognitively impaired elderly. The face-hand test was more specific with less false positives, but also less sensitive because of more false negatives. Basavaraju et al. also noted a bilateral palmomental reflex and extinction in the face-hand test as normal concomitants of aging. In contrast, a unilateral positive palmomental reflex was significantly present in elderly patients with focal neurological damage.

Jenkyn et al. (1977) included younger and delirious patients in their study, and also tested many more primitive reflexes. Using independent results from the Halstead-Reitan battery as the criterion, they found false negative rates less than 60 percent for seven of the reflexes described in Appendix E. Nuchocephalic; Glabellar blink; Suck; Upgaze and Downgaze; Visual tracking; Lateral gaze impersistence; and Paratonia of arms or legs. When three mental status questions were included as part of a screening battery, 64% of mildly, 96% of moderately, and 100% of markedly impaired subjects were correctly predicted, with only 16% false negatives. From the perspective of comparability to the demographics of a general oncology population, this type of screening battery appears particularly promising.

CONCLUSIONS

There is clearly a need for brief, easily administered mental status examinations to detect cognitive impairment due to cancer and the effects of its treatment. In addition to validly measuring cognitive impairment—and not educational, social, or examiner variation—such examinations should be both sensitive in identifying significant deficits and specific in demonstrating their absence. However, especially for the purpose of early detection and treatment of reversible causes of organic mental syndromes, reliability and sensitivity are favored over validity and specificity.

Assessing higher intellectual functioning should be a routine and repetitive component of caring for cancer patients. Abbreviated screening devices should be considered only a preliminary approach to further mental status, physical and laboratory evaluations. Moreover, results from even the most valid of clinical tests for higher intellectual functioning must be interpreted with caution; a thorough knowledge of the patient's premorbid personality and level of function along with knowledge of the differential diagnosis of disturbances causing cognitive impairment are essential for understanding and interpreting bedside testing. A major limitation of standardized screening measures is that they are not free-standing, and cannot be considered apart from other aspects of a patient's evaluation. Thus, although screening mental status exams can be administered by paraprofessionals, interpretation requires training and experience. In addition to improved sensitivity for the presence of organic mental syndromes in cancer patients and improved training in the observational skills necessary for performing a reliable mental status examination, ratings of cognitive abilities should be obtained from more than one observer and include family members' observations.

One criticism of many tests that measure cognition is that they primarily identify gross cognitive changes which are obvious anyway; more urgently needed are improved methods for detecting mild or subtle delirium. The hyperactive patient who is argumentative and combative at one extreme and the quietly stuporous patient who slips into deepening levels of unconsciousness are both fairly easy to diagnose as suffering from delirium because of their obviously altered levels of activity. The average individual whose symptoms are primarily reflected in exaggerated personality traits or affect, or whose diagnosis is not at all so blatant need reliable, repeatable tests. In selecting mental status questions or screens for use in cancer patients, it is important to bear in mind that most of the validity/reliability checks on those measures were done to distinguish psychiatric patients from organic mental syndrome patients, or demented elderly patients from depressed or normal elderly patients. Different results could be reasonably expected in testing cognitively impaired cancer patients from cognitively intact, non-psychiatrically disordered cancer patients.

Several investigators (King, 1982; Meehl & Rosen, 1955) have pointed out that in establishing the validity of diagnostic tests it is important to consider the base rates of the conditions in question. As the prevalence of cognitive impairment increases, improving the accuracy of a test provides more gain. In selecting tests with improved accuracy, however, tests with higher false positive rates are preferable to those with higher false negative rates. This is because of the generally more substantial consequence of failing to detect a potentially reversible problem compared to unnecessarily investigating a non-existent problem. Nevertheless, it emphasizes the importance of more research on the differential rates of cognitive impairment in different cancers and of separating the accuracy of a test from its practical value.

In summary, four major principles of cognitive assessment of cancer patients can be extracted from current knowledge. First, most tests are dependent on a patient's education and intelligence, so that these factors must be considered in the interpretation of any test result. Second, single-item tests and those that are visually dependent are generally to be avoided as they can result in false positives or in inappropriate security from false negative findings. Third, there are serious limitations to all methods of cognitive assessment, but by knowing these and using the same battery or screen routinely and repeatedly, clinicians can maximize the value of the method they use. Finally, and most important, those caring for cancer patients should both increase their awareness for the potential of cognitive impairment and assume some reversibility until further efforts prove otherwise.

REFERENCES

American Psychiatric Association. (1980). *Diagnostic and statistical manual of mental disorders* (3rd ed.). Washington, DC: Author.

Andreasen, N. (1977). Reliability of proverbs: Interpretation to assess mental status. *Comprehensive Psychiatry, 18,* 465–473.

Anthony, J.C., LeResche, L.A., von Korff, M.R., Niaz, U., & Folstein M.F. (1985). Screening for delirium on a general medical ward: The tachistoscope and a global accessibility rating. *General Hospital Psychiatry, 7,* 36–42.

Anthony, J.C., LeResche, L., Niaz, U., von Korff, M.R., & Folstein, M.F. (1982). Limits of the mini-mental state as a screening test for dementia and delirium among hospital patients. *Psychological Medicine, 12,* 397–408.

Basavaraju, N.G., Silverstone, F.A., Libow, L.S., & Paraskevas, K. (1981). Primitive reflexes and perceptual sensory tests in the elderly—their usefulness in dementia. *Journal of Chronic Diseases, 34,* 367–377.

Bender, L. (1938). A visual motor gestalt test and its clinical uses. *American Orthopsychiatric Association Research Monographs, 3.*

Bender, M.B. (1975). The incidence and type of perceptual deficiencies in the aged. In W.S. Fields (Ed.), *Neurological and sensory disorders in the elderly* (pp. 15–31). New York: Stratton Intercontinental Book Corporation.

Benton, A.L. (1963). *The revised visual retention test: Clinical and experimental applications.* New York: The Psychological Coporation.

Blessed, G., Tomlinson, B.E., & Roth, M. (1968). The association between quantitative measures of dementia and of senile change in the cerebral grey matter of elderly subjects. *British Journal of Psychiatry, 114,* 797–811.

Bond, J., Brooks, P., Carstairs, V., & Giles, L. (1980). The reliability of a Survey Psychiatric Assessment Schedule for the elderly. *British Journal of Psychiatry, 137,* 148–162.

Brilliant, P., & Gynther, M. (1963). Relationships between performance on three tests for organicity and selected patient variables. *Jounal of Consulting Psychology, 27,* 474–479.

Brink, T.L. (1981). Self-ratings of memory versus psychometric ratings of memory and hypochondriasis. *Journal of the American Geriatrics Society, 29,* 537–538.

Brinks, T.L., Bryant, J., Catalano, M.L., Janakes, C., & Oliveira, C. (1979). Senile confusion: Assessment with a new stimulus recognition test. *Journal of the American Geriatrics Society, 27,* 126–129.

Conn, H.O. (1977). Trailmaking and number-connection tests in the assessment of mental state in portal systemic encephalopathy. *Digestive Diseases, 22,* 541–550.

Cresswell, D.L., & Lanyon, R.I. (1981). Validation of a screening battery for psychogeriatric assessment. *Journal of Gerontology, 36,* 435–440.

Denham, M.J., & Jefferys, P.M. (1972). Routine mental assessment in elderly patients. *Modern Geriatrics, 2,* 2–8.

Dick, J.P., Guloff, R.J., Steward, A., Blackstock, J., Bielawska, C., Paul, E.A., & Marsden, C.D. (1984). Mini-mental state examination in neurological patients. *Journal of Neurology, Neurosurgery and Psychiatry, 47,* 496–499.

Eslinger, P.J., Damasio, A.R., Benton, A.L., & Van Allen, M. (1985). Neuropsychologic detection of abnormal mental decline in older persons. *Journal of the American Medical Association, 253,* 670–674.

Fillenbaum, G.G. (1980). Comparison of two brief tests of organic brain impairment, the MSQ and the Short Portable MSQ. *Journal of the American Geriatrics Society, 28,* 381–384.

Fink, M., Green, M., & Bender, M.B. (1952). The face-hand test as a diagnostic sign of organic mental syndrome. *Neurology, 2,* 46–58.

Folstein, M.F., Folstein, S.E., & McHugh, P.R. (1975). Mini-mental state: A practical method for grading the cognitive state of patients for the clinician. *Journal of Psychiatric Research, 12,* 189–198.

Folstein, M.F., Fetting, J.H., Lobo, A., Unaiza, N., & Capozzoli, K.D. (1984). Cognitive assessment of cancer patients. *Cancer, 53,* (Suppl.), 2250–2257.

Fries, J.F. (1980). Aging, natural death, and the compression of morbidity. *New England Journal of Medicine, 303,* 130–135..

Gehi, M., Strain, J.J., Weltz, N., & Jacobs, J. (1980). Is there a need for admission and discharge cognitive screening for the medically ill? *General Hospital Psychiatry, 2,* 186–191.

Goodwin, J.M., Goodwin, J.S., & Kellner, R. (1979). Psychiatric symptoms in disliked medical patients. *Journal of the American Medical Association, 241,* 1117–1120.

Graham, F.K., & Kendall, B.S. (1960). Memory-for-designs test: Revised general manual. *Perceptual and Motor Skills, 11,* 147–188.

Helzer, J.E. (1981). The use of a structured diagnostic interview for routine evaluations. *Journal of Nervous and Mental Disorders, 169,* 45–49.

Horne, R.L., Evans, F.J., & Orne, M.T. (1982). Random number generation, psychopathology, and therapeutic change. *Archives of General Psychiatry, 39,* 680–683.

Irving, G., Robinson, R.A., & McAdam, W. (1970). The validity of some cognitive tests in the diagnosis of dementia. *British Journal of Psychiatry, 117,* 149–156.

Isaacs, B., & Kennie, A.T. (1973). The set test as an aid to the detection of dementia in old people. *British Journal of Psychiatry, 123,* 467–470.

Jacobs, J.W., Bernhard, M.R., Delgado, A., & Strain, J.J. Screening for organic mental syndromes in the medically ill. *Annals of Internal Medicine, 86,* 40–46.

Jenkyn, L.R., Walsh, D.B., Culver, C.M., & Reeves, A.G. (1977). Clinical signs in diffuse cerebral dysfunction. *Journal of Neurology, Neurosurgery and Psychiatry, 40,* 956–966.

Kahn, R.L., Goldfarb, A.I., Pollack, M., & Peck, A. (1960). Brief objective measures for the determination of mental status in the aged. *American Journal of Psychiatry, 117,* 326–328.

Kaplan, R. (1984). Substantive and methodological issues in a rating of cognitive and psychological function in multiple sclerosis. *Acta Neurologica Scandinavica, 101,* (Suppl.), 21–28.

Katzman, R., Brown, T., Fuld, P., Peck, A., Shecter, R., & Schimmel, H., (1983). Validation of a short Orientation, Memory Concentration Test of cognitive impairment. *American Journal of Psychiatry, 140,* 734–739.

Kaufman, D.M., Weinberger, M., Strain, J.J., & Jacobs, J.W. (1979). Detection of cognitive deficits by a brief mental status examination: The cognitive capacity screening examination, a reappraisal and a review. *General Hospital Psychiatry, 1,* 247–254.

Keller, M.B., & Manschreck, T.C. (1981). The bedside mental status examination—reliability and validity. *Comprehensive Psychiatry, 22,* 500–511.

King, M.C. (1982). Additional problems with the bedside mental status examination: A note on Keller and Manschreck. *Comprehensive Psychiatry, 23,* 386–387.

Kurucz, J., Feldmar, G., & Werner, W. (1979). Prosopoaffective agnosia associated with chronic organic brain syndrome. *Journal of American Geriatrics Society, 27,* 91–95.

Levine, P.M., Silberfarb, P.M., & Lipowski, Z.J. (1978). Mental disorders in cancer patients: A study of 100 psychiatric referrals. *Cancer, 43,* 1385–1391.

Lezak, M.D. (1976). *Neuropsychological assessment.* New York: Oxford University Press.

Lipowski, Z.J. (1978). Organic brain syndromes: A reformulation. *Comprehensive Psychiatry, 19,* 309–322.

Lipowski, Z.J. (1980). Delirium updated. *Comprehensive Psychiatry, 21,* 190–196.

Manning, R.T. (1982). The serial sevens test. *Archives of Internal Medicine, 142,* 1192.

Matarazzo, J.D. (1972). *Wechsler's measurement and appraisal of adult intelligence* (5th ed). Baltimore: Williams & Wilkins Co.

McEvoy, J.P. (1981). Organic brain syndromes. *Annals of Internal Medicine, 95,* 212–220.

Meadows, P.M., & Evans, A.E. (1976). Effects of chemotherapy on the central nervous system. *Cancer, 37,* 1079–1085.

Meehl, P.M., & Rosen, A. Antecedent probability and the efficiency of psychometric signs, patterns, or cutting scores. *Psychological Bulletin, 52,* 194–216.

Melges, F.T. (1975). Mental status examination. In C.P. Rosenbaum, & J.E. Beebe (Eds.), *Psychiatric treatment: Crisis/clinic/consultation* (pp. 532–533). New York: McGraw-Hill.

Oxman, T.E., & Silberfarb, P.M. (1980). Serial cognitive testing in cancer patients receiving chemotherapy. *American Journal of Psychiatry, 137,* 1263–1265.

Paulker, N.E., Folstein, M.F., & Moran, T.H. (1978). The clinical utility of the hand-held tachistoscope. *Journal of Nervous and Mental Disorders, 166,* 126–153.

Pfeiffer, E. (1975). A short portable mental status questionnaire for the assessment of organic brain deficit in elderly patients. *Journal of the American Geriatrics Society, 23,* 433–441.

Rabins, P.V., & Folstein, M.F. (1982). Delirium and dementia: Diagnostic criteria and fatality rates. *British Journal of Psychiatry, 140,* 149–153.

Raven, J.C. (1958). *Guide to using the mill hill vocabulary scale and the progressive matrices scales.* London: H.K. Lewis.

Reich, J.H. (1981). Proverbs and the modern mental status exam. *Comprehensive Psychiatry, 22,* 528–531.

Reitan, R.M. (1977). A research program on the psychological effects of brain lesions in human beings. In N. Ellis (Ed.), *International review of mental retardation: Vol. 1.* New York: Academic Press.

Reitan, R.M., & Davison, L.A. (1974). *Clinical neuropsychology: Current status and applications.* New York: Wiley and Sons.

Reitan, R.M. (1958). Validity of the trail making test as an indicator of organic brain damage. *Perceptual and Motor Skills, 8,* 271–276.

Roe, P.F. (1982). Prognostic value of the abbreviated mental status questionnaire. *Gerontology, 28,* 252–257.

Sadavoy, J., & Reiman-Sheldon, E. (1983). General hospital geriatric psychiatric treatment: A follow-up study. *Journal of the American Geriatrics Society, 31,* 200–205.

Silberfarb, P.M. (1983). Chemotherapy and cognitive defects in cancer patients. *Annual Review of Medicine, 34,* 35–46.

Silberfarb, P.M., Philibert, D., & Levine, P.M. (1980). Psychosocial aspects of neoplastic disease: II. Affective and cognitive effects of chemotherapy in cancer patients. *American Journal of Psychiatry, 137,* 597–601.

Strub, R.L., & Black, F.W. (1977). *The mental status examination in neurology.* Philadelphia: FA Davis Company.

Talland, G.A. (1965). *Deranged memory: A psychonomic study of the amnesia syndrome.* New York: Academic Press.

Taylor, M.A., Abrams, R., Faber, R., & Almy, G. (1980). Cognitive tasks in the mental status examination. *Journal of Nervous and Mental Diseases, 168,* 167–170.

Tsai, L., & Tsuang, M.T. (1979). The Mini-mental state test and computerized tomography. *American Journal of Psychiatry, 136,* 436–439.

Webster, J.S., Scott, R.R., Nunn, B., McNeer, M.F., & Varnell, N. (1984). A brief neuropsychological screening procedure that assesses left and right hemispheric function. *Journal of Clinical Psychology, 40,* 237–40.

Wechsler, D. (1972). *Measurement and appraisal of adult intelligence* (3rd ed.). New York: Brunner/Mazel.

Whybrow, P.C., & Spencer, R.F. (1969). Changing characteristics of psychiatric consultation in a university hospital. *Canadian Psychiatric Association Journal, 14,* 259–266.

Wolber, G., Romaniuk, M., Eastman, E., & Robinson, C. (1984). Validity of the short portable mental status questionnaire with elderly psychiatric patients. *Journal of Consulting and Clinical Psychology, 52,* 712–713.

Yates, A.J. (1966). Psychological deficit. *Annual Review of Psychology, 17,* 111–144.

APPENDIX A

The Mental Status Examination: Questions for Assessment of Cognitive Function (Matarazzo, 1972; Melges, 1975; Strub and Black, 1977)

COGNITIVE FUNCTION	*SUGGESTED TECHNIQUE*
ORIENTATION	What day of the week is it? What is the date? What room, floor, wing, and building are we in?
MEMORY	To test recent memory, give the patient three unrelated words (e.g., table, eighty-nine, honesty) to remember for five minutes. Ask the patient to recite them immediately to be sure he or she heard them. For remote memory ask for the patient's birthdate or mother's maiden name.
ATTENTION AND CONCEN-TRATION	*Digit Span* The patient is asked to repeat increasing series of numbers forward (e.g. 5,3,7; 1,5,8,3,; 2,9,6,4,1) and then another increasing series backward. The examiner should say the digits at a rate of one per second and should drop his or her voice with the last digit to signal the end. If the patient makes an error on any series, one more series of the same number of digits should be given, stopping after two failures at any given number of digits. Less than five digits forward and three backward or a discrepancy greater than two between the number of digits forward and

backward is suggestive of an organic mental syndrome.

Serial 7s or 3s
The patient is asked to subtract aloud (without writing) 7 from 100 and then from each subsequent answer. Observation is made for increased effort and time and forgetting what the task was. For repeated use, the patient should be asked to start at numbers other than 100 (e.g., 99 or 101). If the patient cannot do this task at all, serial 3s should be used, or the patient should be asked to start at a given number, count by ones and stop at another given number.

ABSTRACTION

Proverbs
The patient is told, "Do you know what a proverb is? It is a saying about people only using objects or other living things. For example, what do the following tell us about human nature: Don't count your chickens before they are hatched; Rome wasn't built in a day; A stitch in time saves nine; A drowning man will clutch at a straw?" Assessment of a patient's response is based on performing abstraction at the time of the examination rather then from memory. Rate the quality of the patient's response as concrete, semi-abstract, or abstract. The average patient should provide abstract interpretation to at least two proverbs and semiabstract responses to the other two. Be sure to ask about the patient's educational level to help in interpretation of answers.

Similarities

The capacity to find general principles or similarities in two overtly different objects or terms is tested by asking the patient to "tell me how the following pairs of objects are similar, what do they have in common: cat and mouse; paper and coal; mountain and lake; horse and apple?" A response is considered concrete and suggestive of lower intelligence or impaired abstraction when the response reflects a property of only one member of the pair, is a difference, or unrelated to either member.

CONSTRUC-
TIONAL ABILITY   On separate sheets of unlined paper, draw a horizontal diamond, a two-dimensional cross, and a three dimensional cube. Then ask the patient to draw, without copying, simple pictures of a clock and a house in perspective.

APPENDIX B

Brief Cognitive Screening Examinations

Name   *Description and References*

Analogue Scales   Global impression of examiner is marked on a line which can be measured. Anchoring descriptions are provided for the extremes. Rating made by trained observer after 2 minute interaction (Anthony, LeResche, von Korff, Niaz & Folstein, 1985; Folstein et al., 1984)

Bender Visual Motor Gestalt Test	Nine simple designs are presented on cards to the patient for copying, one at a time. The type and frequency of errors are noted (Bender, 1938; Brilliant & Gynther, 1963)
Benton Visual Retention Test	The subject must draw a geometric design from memory, requiring short-term retention and recall as well as spatio-constructive abilities. The test can be altered by using shorter card exposures. Performance is scored by the number of cards correctly reproduced and by the number of errors. (Benton, 1963; Brilliant & Gynther, 1963)
Cognitive Capacity Screening Exam	Thirty questions testing orientation, memory, attention, calculation, and abstraction. Requires ability to rapidly shift from one type of item to another (Jacobs et al., 1977; Gehi, Strain, Weltz & Jacobs, 1980)
Graham Kendall Memory for Designs	Copying of a series of simple geometric figures from immediate memory after seeing figure for 5 seconds. Raw scores of number and types of errors can be adjusted for age and IQ (Graham and Kendall, 1960; Wolber, Romaniuk, Eastman & Robinson, 1984)
Information-Memory-Concentration Mental Status Test	Information is tested by orientation and recognition of persons; memory by historical and personal events and

	by five minute recall of a name and address; concentration by counting forwards and backwards from 20 and saying the months in reverse order (Blessed, Tomlinson & Roth, 1968)
Mental Status Questionnaire	Ten questions concerning orientation to time place, and person, and the current and past President (Bond, Brooks, Carstairs & Giles, 1980; Brink, 1981; Brink et al., 1979; Cresswell & Lanyon, 1981; Fillenbaum, 1980; Kahn et al., 1960)
Mental Status Questionnaire	British version of ten questions of orientation, recognition of 2 people, counting backwards 20-1, Prime Minister, and recall of a 7 word sentence (Bond et al., 1980; Denham & Jefferys, 1972)
Mini-Mental Status	Divided into two sections, the first covers orientation, memory, and attention, and the second tests language and constructional abilities (Anthony et al., 1982, 1985; Folstein et al., 1975; Folstein et al., 1984)
Modified Mental Status Questionnaire	Ten questions used by Denham and Jefferys plus 6 practical tests such as copying a pattern of matchsticks arranged in a zig-zag and triangle (Roe, 1982)
Orientation-Memory-Concentration Test	Shortened 6 item version of Information-Memory-Concentration Mental Status. Includes 3 orientation ques-

tions, a phrase to remember, counting backwards 20-1, and saying the months in reverse order (Katzman, Brown, Fuld, Peck, Shecter & Schimmel, 1983)

Short Portable
Mental Status
Questionnaire

Pfeiffer's modification of the Mental Status Questionnaire. Differs in that scoring reflects race and education (Pfeiffer, 1975; Fillenbaum, 1980; Sadavoy & Reiman-Sheldon, 1983)

Stimulus
Recognition Test

Ten trials of presentation of stimuli (e.g., digits, shapes, objects, words, letters). Patient is to tell examiner to stop when the same stimulus is presented again (Brink et al., 1979; Brink, 1981; Wolber et al., 1984)

Random Number
Generation

Patients are told to randomly say 100 numbers aloud using the numbers 1-10 inclusive in time with a metronome. A randomization index is computed. Patients with organic mental syndrome produce less random series (Horne, Evans & Orne, 1982)

Raven's Progressive
Matrices

A series of printed designs from each of which a part has been removed. The missing portion is presented in a series of alternatives. Developed as a measure of intelligence (Raven, 1958; Irving, Robinson & McAdam, 1970)

Set Test

The patient is asked to name 10 colors, fruits, towns and animals, and is given one point for each. (Issacs & Kinnie, 1984)

Tachistoscope   Hand held version which is a camera shutter with adjustable exposure times. Patient is asked to look in and identify a simple stimulus (Anthony et al., 1985; Paulker, Folstein & Moran, 1978)

Trail Making Test   A timed test requiring connection of numbers and letters in alternating ascending sequence (Conn, 1977; Oxman & Silberfarb, 1980)

APPENDIX C

Mini-Mental State Exam
(Folstein, et al., 1975)

Maximum Score	Score		

ORIENTATION

5	( )	What is the (year) (season) (day) (month)?
5	( )	Where are we: (state) (country) (town) (hospital) (floor)?

REGISTRATION

3	( )	Name 3 objects: 1 second to say each. Then ask the patient all 3 after you have said them. Give 1 point for each correct answer. Then repeat them until he learns all 3. Count trials and record.

TRIALS

ATTENTION AND CALCULATION

5	( )	Serial 7s. 1 point for each correct. Stop after 5 answers. Alternatively spell "world" backwards.

RECALL

3   ( )   Ask for 3 objects repeated above. Give 1 point for each correct.

LANGUAGE

9   ( )   Name a pencil, and watch (2 points). Repeat the following "No ifs, ands, or buts." (1 point) Follow a 3-stage command: "Take a paper in your right hand, fold it in half, and put it on the floor." (3 points) Read and obey the following: "Close your eyes" (1 point) Write a sentence (1 point) Copy design (1 point)

TOTAL SCORE Assess level of consciousness along a continuum:

Alert   Drowsy   Stupor   Coma

APPENDIX D

Cognitive Capacity Screening Examination
(Jacobs et al., 1977)

1. What day of the week is this?   _____
2. What month?   _____
3. What day of month?   _____
4. What year?   _____
5. What place is this?   _____
6. Repeat the numbers 8 7 2.   _____
7. Say them backwards.   _____
8. Repeat these numbers 6 3 7 1.   _____
9. Listen to these numbers 6 9 4. Count 1 through 10 out loud, then repeat 6 9 4. (Help if needed. Then use 5 7 3).   _____
10. Listen to these numbers 8 1 4 3. Count 1 through 10 out loud, then repeat 8 1 4 3.   _____

11. Beginning with Sunday, say the days of the
    week backwards.   _____
12. 9 + 3 is   _____
13. Add 6 to the previous answer (or "to 12")   _____
14. Take away 5 ("from 18").   _____
15. The opposite of fast is slow.
    The opposite of up is   _____
16. The opposite of large is   _____
17. The opposite of hard is   _____
18. An orange and a banana are both fruits.
    Red and blue are both   _____
19. A penny and a dime are both   _____
20. What were those words I asked you to
    remember? (HAT)   _____
21. (CAR)   _____
22. (TREE)   _____
23. (TWENTY-SIX)   _____
24. Take away 7 from 100, then take away 7
    from what is left and keep going: 100 − 7 is   _____
25. Minus 7   _____
26. Minus 7   _____
27. Minus 7   _____
28. Minus 7   _____
29. Minus 7   _____
30. Minus 7   _____

TOTAL CORRECT
(maximum = 30) _____ Occupation:
Education: Age: Estimated intelligence (based on
education, occupation, and history, not test score):

    Below average   Average   Above average

Patient was:
Cooperative   Uncooperative   Depressed   Lethargic   Other

APPENDIX E

Primitive Reflexes in Diffuse Cerebral Dysfunction
(Jenkyn et al., 1977; Basavaraju et al., 1981)

Reflex	*Description*
Nuchocephalic	Normally the head turns when the shoulders are turned in a standing patient whose eyes are closed.
Paratonia	Normally when resting muscle tone is tested by passive extension and flexion of the arms and legs there should be no opposition to the examiner's movements after instructions to relax.
Palmomental	Normally, when the thenar eminence of the patient's hand is given a noxious stroke with the examiner's thumb nail, there will be no contraction of the ipsilateral mentalis chin muscle on less then five of ten consecutive strokes.
Grasp	Normally when told not to do so a patient will not grasp the examiner's fingers when they stroke the palmar surface of the patient's hand. The addition of a distracting task such as spell "world" backwards, can be used to increase the appearance of the abnormally disinhibited reflex.
Suck	Normally there is no pursing or sucking motion of the patient's lips when the examiner firmly places the knuckle of a finger between the patient's lips.
Glabellar blink	Normally reflex closure of the eyelids to tapping of the glabellar region is inhibited after three taps and the lids remain open.

Decreased upward and/or lateral gaze	Normally a patient's eyes will deviate more than 5–7mm from the midposition when he is asked to follow the examiner's finger as it is moved to all extremes of vertical and horizontal gaze.
Lateral gaze impersistence	Normally a patient can maintain his gaze on the examiner's finger at approximately a 45 degree angle in the horizontal plane for 30 seconds.
Visual tracking	Normally a patient's eyes will smoothly (without irregular, hesitant, jerking saccades) follow the examiner's finger as it moves between both extremes of horizontal gaze.

Patient and Family Satisfaction
With Care for the Terminally Ill

Ron D. Hays
Sharon Arnold

ABSTRACT. The importance of patient satisfaction as an outcome of medical care for the terminally ill prompted a review and evaluation of the literature. We begin by offering a conceptual framework for patient satisfaction. Then, we summarize the empirical studies addressing patient and family satisfaction with care for the terminally ill. Finally, we provide guidelines for patient satisfaction assessment and evaluate the empirical research in accord with these guidelines.

An increasing emphasis on patients as consumers of services in the medical marketplace underscores the significance of satisfaction assessment as a criterion of the quality of medical care. The extent to which different delivery systems satisfy their patients will be a major determinant of the viability of these systems. Patient and family satisfaction with medical care for the terminally ill is particularly important; in contrast to the typical medical focus on prolonging life and curing disease, treatment for the terminally ill demands an emphasis on palliative care. It has been suggested that health care professionals are uncomfortable and have trouble treating the terminally ill because they equate inability to cure illness with failure (Edwardson, 1985). Dying is a taboo topic in our society. When prevention of mortality is no longer perceived possible, the

Ron D. Hays, PhD, is an associate behavioral scientist, The Rand Corporation; Sharon Arnold is a graduate fellow of The Rand UCLA Center for Health Policy Studies. Preparation of this paper was made possible by grants for the National Study of Medical Care Outcomes from the Robert Wood Johnson Foundation and from the Henry J. Kaiser Family Foundation. The opinions expressed are those of the authors and do not necessarily reflect the views of the Sponsors or the Rand Corporation.

Requests for reprints may be sent to Ron D. Hays, Behavioral Sciences Department, The Rand Corporation, 1700 Main Street, Santa Monica, CA 90406.

129

patient tends to be "abandoned by both the health care estab-
lishment and society in general" (Kastenbaum, 1979, p. 189).
It is held to be society's responsibility to maximize the quality
of life of the dying and not abandon them (Aroskar, 1985).

Increasing public concern with quality of life of the dying
patient has resulted in efforts to improve the medical care
provided during the terminal phase of life. Criticism of excessive use of biomedical technology, prolonged course of disease, and unnecessary suffering and pain in terminal care is
being vocalized as the customer's demand for "healthy dying"
(Kastenbaum, 1979). The hospice concept has become very
popular as an alternative to the traditional care received by
the terminal patient. A recent study of the attitudes of seriously ill patients revealed that 80% of those surveyed reported that they would use hospice care if it was made available to them (Rainey, Crane, Breslow, & Ganz, 1984).

The hospice is characterized by (a) care for the individual
rather then treatment of the disease, (b) palliative rather than
curative care, (c) pain control and symptom management as
high priorities, (d) equality between the patient/family and
health care professionals, and (e) concern for interpersonal
over technical aspects of medical care (Franco, 1985; Kastenbaum, 1979; Vandenbos, DeLeon, & Pallak, 1982). The hospice considers the patient/family as the *unit* of care (Smith,
1984), implying that the needs of the family as well as the
patient are equally important. Hospice professionals are known
to evaluate family members to insure that *their* psychosocial
needs are met. Some have even suggested that the family is the
primary provider and recipient of hospice care, and that "professional care providers should defer to the judgment of the
patient and family" (Bass, 1985, p. 309).

Hospice care emerged as an alternative means of treatment
because of dissatisfaction with traditional medical care for the
dying patient (Edwardson, 1985; Paradis, 1984). In view of
the strong interest in the hospice philosophy of patient care
and its therapeutic potential, any evaluation of terminal care,
whether hospice or traditional medical care, needs to examine
the satisfaction of patients and their families with that care.
The demand for hospice care has grown because of its emphasis on the satisfaction of the patient and family, but there is
also evidence that hospice care may be less expensive than

conventional care, especially in the last month of life (Hannah & O'Donnell, 1984; Mor & Kidder, 1985).

The consequent importance of the terminally ill patient and family's satisfaction with the medical care they receive prompted the present review. We begin by offering our conceptual framework of patient satisfaction. Then the results of studies of patient and family satisfaction with terminal care are summarized. Next, important issues in patient satisfaction assessment are discussed and the research on patient and family satisfaction with care for the terminally ill is reviewed with respect to these issues.

CONCEPTUALIZATION OF PATIENT SATISFACTION

Empirical studies of patient satisfaction with medical care have tended to be conducted without an explicit conceptual framework (Pascoe, 1983). Careful theoretical analysis is needed in order to elucidate the importance of patient satisfaction with medical care. We provide a social-psychological theory of patient satisfaction that is useful for understanding different approaches to patient satisfaction assessment and the recommendations we offer for future research.

Patient satisfaction has been operationalized in varying ways by different investigators. However, there is a consensus that it is, at least in part, an "attitude" (Linder-Pelz, 1982; Risser, 1975). A prevailing model of attitudes in the 1940s, 1950s, and 1960s included three major components: *affect, cognitive* (beliefs), and *conative* (behavioral intentions) (Rosenberg & Hovland, 1960). This attitudinal trilogy is still widely endorsed (see Bagozzi & Burnkrant, 1985; Dillon & Kumar, 1985). However, we favor Ajzen and Fishbein's (1980) operationalization of attitudes as the *affective* component of the trilogy. According to Ajzen and Fishbein (1980), attitudes are affective responses (general feelings of favorableness or unfavorableness) to persons, objects, and concepts. Beliefs in combination with the value or importance of the outcomes associated with the beliefs lead to the formation of attitudes (affective responses). In turn, attitudes and subjective norms influence behavioral intentions and behavior. Thus, affect, beliefs, and behavioral intentions are conceptually distinct but interrelated concepts.

Hays (1985) presented an integrated theory of behavior that expands the Ajzen-Fishbein framework. A schematic representation of this theory is given in Figure 1. According to the theory, whether or not a patient exhibits the behavior to utilize a system of medical care is the result of four direct effects: (1) the patient's intention to use that system of care when care is needed (Behavioral Intention); (2) the patient's prior utilization of services of the system (Former Behavior); (3) the patient's satisfaction with care received (Patient Satisfaction); and (4) the patient's internal control over utilization (Internal-External Behavioral Locus Of Control). Patient satisfaction, hence, is depicted as a significant predictor of utilization. By patient satisfaction we refer to the patient's positive or negative evaluation of medical care (i.e., the degree to which the patient is satisfied or dissatisfied with care received). Beliefs about aspects of medical care (e.g, "The doctors at System X are competent and well-trained") weighted by the value or perceived importance of the outcomes associated with these beliefs ("It is very important to me to have competent and well-trained doctors") determine patient satisfaction with medical care (Linder-Pelz, 1982). Of course, patient satisfaction is a function of other salient beliefs and their associated values or importance in addition to the belief noted above. Thus, patient satisfaction is a function of all beliefs about specific features of care. Similarly, intention to utilize a system of care is a function of satisfaction and whether important others feel the patient should utilize that system of care (Perceived Norms Toward Behavior).[1]

SUMMARY OF RESEARCH ON SATISFACTION WITH TERMINAL CARE

Surveys of patient satisfaction with medical care have burgeoned in recent years to the extent that satisfaction is now a major subcategory of research in the field of social psychology and medicine. Ware, Davies-Avery, and Stewart (1978) identified over 100 articles on patient satisfaction in their review of 25 years of work in the field. In a more recent review of patient satisfaction research, Pascoe (1983) cited nearly 200 different references. Although at least 4000 publications on death and

Figure 1

Theory Of Patient Satisfaction And Medical Care Utilization

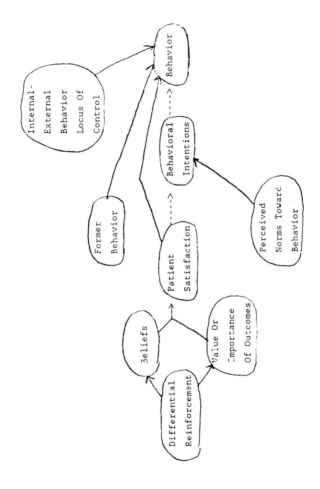

dying are available (see Fulton, 1977), almost all of the research reviewed by Ware et al. (1978) and Pascoe (1983) were
surveys of patient satisfaction among ambulatory care patients
or general household respondents. Very few studies of the
satisfaction of terminally ill patients and their families have
been published (McCusker, 1984). Table 1 lists all the published empirical research we located pertaining to patient and
family satisfaction with terminal care.[2] The paucity of studies in
Table 1 is ironic given the overwhelming importance of satisfaction in terminal medical care.

In a study of 74 children with cancer (Barbarin & Chesler,
1984), ratings along seven dimensions of care were made by

Table 1

Studies Of Patient And Family Satisfaction
With Care For The Terminally Ill

Investigators	Respondent	Sample Size	Dimensions Of Satisfaction	Data Medium
Barbarin & Chesler (1984)	(S)	74	(COM, GEN, INF, INT, TEC)	(I,S)
Barzelai (1981)	(S)	20	(INF, PM)	(S)
Creek (1982)	(S)	45	(GEN, INT, PM)	(S)
Hannan & O'Donnell (1984)	(S)	350	(INT, TEC)	(S,T)
Kane, Klein, Bernstein, Rothenberg, & Wales (1985); Wales, Kane, Robbins, Bernstein, & Krasnow (1983)	(P,S)	115, 135	(GEN, INT, INV, PE, PM, TEC)	(I)
McCusker (1984)	(P,S) (S)	102, 111 96	(AV, COM, CON, GEN, INT, INV, PM, TEC)	(I,S)

Note. Letters in parentheses represent the following: Respondent:
P=patient, S=significant other; Dimensions Of Satisfaction:
AV=availability of care, COM=communication, CON=continuity, GEN=general
satisfaction, INF=information giving, INT=interpersonal, INV=involvement
in care/treatment decisions, PM=pain/symptom management, PE=physical
environment, TEC=technical care; Data Gathering Medium: I=interview,
S=self-administered questionnaire, T=telephone.

trained coders on a *Poor* to *Excellent* response scale based on the responses given by the children's parents during an extensive open-ended interview. These ratings included satisfaction with interpersonal care (communication, empathy, warmth and concern), technical care (staff's knowledge and skill), information giving, conflict resolution, and the family's participation in care. Global or general satisfaction with care was assessed with a composite index derived from parental self-reported ratings of anger, respect, liking, tenseness, and support. Although central tendency (means) and variability statistics were not reported in the paper, Barbarin and Chesler (1984) did indicate that ratings on the specific dimensions of care accounted for 37% of the variance in the global satisfaction index.

In another study, 20 surviving relatives (spouse, children, mother, or girlfriend) of patients who had been in a hospice program (for longer than two weeks) completed a 21-item questionnaire assessing perceptions of the hospice experience (Barzelai, 1981). The wording of the items was not indicated, but the questionnaire appeared to assess global perceptions about the effectiveness of hospice care. Relief from pain, relief from other physical problems, relief from anxiety (both patient and significant other), satisfaction with information giving, and whether or not the respondent would recommend the program to a friend or relative were measured. As a result of the hospice team intervention, 82% of the relatives reported that the patients received relief from pain most or all of the time, 88% reported some relief from physical problems, and 64% reported relief from anxiety (89% of the significant others experienced relief from anxiety). All of the respondents indicated that they would recommend the hospice to a friend or relative. However, dissatisfaction with information giving by the physician can be inferred by the fact that only 45% of the respondents reported that the physician was a good source of information.

Creek (1982) studied satisfaction with hospice care by asking care givers (spouse, adult child, or significant other non-family member) of hospice patients to report on satisfaction with care. Caregivers were asked to report their own and the family's satisfaction with the physician, nursing care, social worker, and the pain medications given the patient. Satisfaction was assessed on a scale with possible responses ranging from 100 percent dissatisfied to 100 percent satisfied. Respondents were asked to place an "X" on the location of the scale that represented their satisfaction level for each of the features of care rated. Average satisfaction scores for caregivers and family exceeded 90% for nursing care, the social worker, and effectiveness of pain medication. Mean satisfaction with the physician was 75% for caregivers and 78% for the family (as reported by the caregiver).

As part of the evaluation of hospices in the New York State Demonstration Program, Hannan and O'Donnell (1984) measured the satisfaction of 350 primary care providers with the care received by patients participating in 12 hospice programs. The primary care providers were asked about the patient's satisfaction as well as their own satisfaction with the hospice. Satisfaction with nursing services, physician services, pastoral care, therapy services, social services, home health aide services, and volunteer services were evaluated. Respondents used a five-point scale from "Very Satisfied" to "Very Dissatisfied," or rated the item inapplicable. The percentage of satisfied respondents (those reporting that they were "very satisfied" or "satisfied") was quite high across the various features of care, ranging from 84% to 100%. Satisfaction with hospital care of the patient was higher for hospital-based programs than community-based programs ($p < .05$).

A satisfaction with interpersonal care scale developed by Ware, Johnston, Davies-Avery, and Brook (1979), a satisfaction with involvement in care scale adopted from the National Cancer Institute's Hospice study (Baker, 1981; cited in Kane, Klein, Bernstein, Rothenberg, & Wales, 1985) and a satisfaction with physical environment scale adopted from McCaffree and Harkins (1976; cited in Kane et al., 1985) were employed in a randomized controlled trial of 115 patients and 135 significant others at the Wadsworth VA Hospice (Kane et al., 1985). No significant difference in satisfaction with physical environment was found between participants in the hospice program and the control group. Hospice patients were significantly more satisfied than control patients with interpersonal care ($p < .004$) and involvement in care ($p < .02$).

Two evaluative studies of patient satisfaction were published by McCusker (1984). One study (Home Care Study) was a randomized controlled trial comparing a health care team treatment approach with an existing community services approach to home care for primarily elderly, chronically ill patients suffering from a variety of illnesses (cancer, stroke, degenerative neurological diseases). The satisfaction of patients and caretakers with the care delivered to the patients was assessed. In the second study (Terminal Care Study), a relative of each of the cancer patients was asked retrospectively about care during the last six months of the patient's life. Satisfaction with availability of care, availability of doctors, continuity of care, technical care, interpersonal care, communication, general satisfaction, involvement in treatment decisions, and pain management were measured in one or both studies using multiple-item scales. Five-point Likert-type response options were used with the satisfaction items.

Average satisfaction levels were about the middle of the possible score range for both patients (n = 102) and caretakers (n = 111) in the Home Care Study. Patients reported higher levels of satisfaction with care received than did the caretakers (p < .01 for general satisfaction and satisfaction with personal qualities of the physician). Postbereavement ratings of general satisfaction, satisfaction with availability of care, freedom from pain, and pain control were statistically higher (p's < .01) for caretakers of patients assigned to the health care team treatment than they were for those assigned to the existing services group. Mean satisfaction levels for relatives (n = 96) of patients in the Terminal Care Study were about the middle of the possible score range.

IMPORTANT ISSUES IN ASSESSING
SATISFACTION WITH TERMINAL CARE

Assessment of patient satisfaction requires attention to the data gathering medium, patient satisfaction item structure, dimensions of satisfaction, construction of multiple-item scales, and reliability and validity of the satisfaction instrument. We discuss and offer suggestions on each of these fundamental measurement issues. The recommendations we provide derive from our experience in developing measures of patient satisfaction for the National Study of Medical Care Outcomes (1985), a longitudinal study which examines patient satisfaction and other outcomes for patients with chronic physical or mental illness, who are receiving care from different specialists and in different systems of care.

Data Gathering Medium

One of the first issues confronted in patient satisfaction assessment is the medium by which the data will be gathered. Information about patient satisfaction may be obtained by self-administered questionnaires, telephone interviews, or by face-to-face interviews. Dillman (1978) provides an excellent source of information about the relative strengths and weaknesses of these different data gathering mediums. Self-administered questionnaires have the strength of lower response bias compared to telephone and face-to-face interviews because respondents are able to answer questions in privacy (responses are made without the presence of a potential evaluator) and at their own pace. They also have the advantage of permitting more detailed questioning of respondents than is permitted when greater time pressures exist, as is the case with telephone and face-to-face interviews. Furthermore, self-administered questionnaires cost from 1/3 to 1/2 as much as telephone and face-to-face interviews. Because of its advantages, the self-administered questionnaire has been used frequently for studies of patient satisfaction.

The self-administered questionnaire may not always be appropriate for studies of satisfaction with terminal care. If the satisfaction of very sick patients is assessed, for example, it may be necessary to conduct face-to-face interviews or combine face-to-face interviewing techniques with self-administered surveys. One of the six studies listed in Table 1 gathered patient satisfaction information from face-to-face interviews only (Kane et al., 1985; Wales, Kane, Robbins, Bernstein, & Krasnow, 1983), two studies used self-administered questionnaires only (Barzelai, 1981; Creek, 1982), two studies used face-to-face interviews and self-administered questionnaires (Barbarin & Chesler, 1984; McCusker, 1984), and one study used telephone interviews combined with self-administered surveys (Hannan & O'Donnell, 1984). The patient questionnaire in McCusker's Home Care Study is a good example of

the need to employ more than just the standard self-administered questionnaire to gather satisfaction data. Because her
patients were very sick and/or disabled, a specially designed
card containing satisfaction response options was handed to
the patients and they were asked to point to their response.
Methodological variations such as the one McCusker employed are particularly needed for assessing satisfaction among
the terminally ill.

Item Structure

Patient satisfaction items have two primary components: an
item stem and a set of response options. The item stem contains a description of the feature of medical care that is being
evaluated; the response options are the choices respondents
are given to indicate their degree of satisfaction. Variations of
these components of item structure are illustrated in the examples provided below.

Example #1: How satisfied are you with the medical care you
have received?

1. Very Satisfied
2. Satisfied
3. Neither Satisfied nor Dissatisfied
4. Dissatisfied
5. Very Dissatisfied

Example #2: The doctors who provide my medical care are
competent and well-trained.

1. Strongly Agree
2. Agree
3. Uncertain
4. Disagree
5. Strongly Disagree

The first example represents a "direct" approach to satisfaction assessment while the second example represents an
"indirect" approach. By direct approach we mean that the
item directly corresponds to the conceptualization of satisfac-

tion as an affective response to medical care. Thus, the direct approach employs items that tap this general response to care received. In contrast, the indirect approach involves assessment of salient beliefs about medical care. As noted in our conceptualization of patient satisfaction, salient beliefs and the value or perceived importance of the outcomes associated with these beliefs determine satisfaction with care. With the indirect approach, satisfaction is estimated by summing across salient beliefs.[3] Patient satisfaction assessment by the direct approach requires fewer items than the indirect approach and allows for a direct summary evaluation of care, but it provides no information about the antecedents of satisfaction or dissatisfaction with care. The indirect approach requires more items to represent a given domain of satisfaction, but allows for more detailed understanding about specific features of medical care.

The direct approach was used in three of the satisfaction studies we reviewed (Barzelai, 1981; Creek, 1982; Hannan & O'Donnell, 1984); the indirect approach was employed in two of the studies (McCusker, 1984; Kane et al., 1985). Barbarin and Chesler (1984) employed an indirect-type strategy in which satisfaction was based on ratings of anger with medical staff, respect for medical system, liking of medical staff, tenseness in relations with medical staff, and helpfulness and support of medical staff.

Two sets of response choices, Satisfaction—Dissatisfaction and Agree—Disagree, are represented in the examples presented above. The choice of response options depends in part on whether a direct or indirect approach to measurement is adopted. That is, the interaction of the item stem with the response options requires consideration. For example, direct measurement of satisfaction can be accomplished using Satisfaction—Dissatisfaction response choices combined with item stems containing general expressions about care received. In contrast, satisfaction may be assessed indirectly by combining Agree—Disagree response options with item stems containing statements about specific features of care.

Another set of response options sometimes used for satisfaction assessment is the "Excellent" to "Poor" choices shown below in Example #3. Trained coders employed response categories similar to these when rating the dimensions of satisfaction in Barbarin and Chesler's (1984) study. Although the "Excellent" to "Poor" response categories have not yet been evaluated extensively, in a recent methodological study of satisfaction with a specific medical encounter we compared this format with an "Extremely Satisfied" to a "Very Dissatisfied" response set (Hays & Ware, forthcoming). Item response format was randomly assigned to respondent: half the sample was administered a survey with the "Excellent" to "Poor" response format and the other half was administered the survey with the "Extremely Satisfied" to "Very Dissatisfied" response format. Respondents who received the "Excellent" to "Poor" format had significantly lower satisfaction scores, greater between-respondent score variability, and ratings which were more highly correlated with behavioral intentions (e.g., intention to recommend the doctor to a friend or return to the doctor) than respondents who received the questionnaire with the "Extremely Satisfied" to "Very Dissatisfied" format. Thus, it is not possible to compare directly the results of studies in which the response choices are varied.

Example #3. How would you rate the medical care you have received?

1. Excellent
2. Very Good
3. Good
4. Fair
5. Poor

The number of categories employed to assess patient satisfaction is another important consideration, because the number of categories will have an effect on the accuracy of measurement. Five response categories were used in each of the above examples, but more or less than five categories could have been employed. Why were five categories selected? Careful consideration of the optimal number of response categories to use for patient satisfaction measurement led Ware, Synder, and Wright (1976a, 1976b) to adopt a five choice continuum. Several studies suggest that about five to seven well-chosen response options provide a lower bound for adequate assessment of a measurement domain (Bollen & Barb, 1981; Johnson & Creech, 1983; Johnson & Dixon, 1984; Lissitz & Green, 1975; Ramsay, 1973). Bollen and Barb (1981) concluded that "at a minimum five or six categories should be used . . . the collapsed variables' correlations become considerably closer to the correlation of continuous variables when at least this number of scale points are available" (p. 238).

Creek (1982) employed a continuous response scale for his satisfaction measures; Barzelai (1981) did not provide enough information for the number of options to be determined: a combination of three-point and five-point self-report items as well as open-ended questions (ratings by trained coders of this information made on a five-point scale) were used to obtain information from parents in Barbarin and Chesler's (1984) study. Six-point scales were used by Hannon and O'Donnell (1984), and Kane et al. (1985), and McCusker (1984) used five-point scales.

Dimensions of Satisfaction

Theoretically, patient satisfaction is a multidimensional concept (Ware, 1981; Ware, et al., 1983). Satisfaction with interpersonal care, communication, technical care, time spent with providers, access/availability/convenience, financial arrangements, and general satisfaction were the dimensions chosen to study patient satisfaction in the National Study Of Medical Care Outcomes (1985). The selection of these dimensions was guided by previous research by Ware and his colleagues (see e.g., Ware, Synder, Wright, & Davies, 1983). Studies of satisfaction with medical care for the terminally ill can profit by assessing these same dimensions. Satisfaction with pain management, which has been included in studies of satisfaction with dental care (Davies & Ware, 1981, 1982), is equally relevant for assessments of satisfaction with terminal care.

Most of the key dimensions of satisfaction with terminal care were represented in the studies we reviewed (see Table 1). Satisfaction with interpersonal care, pain/symptom management, and technical care were the most frequently assessed dimensions of satisfaction. McCusker's (1984) study was more comprehensive than the other studies of patient satisfaction with terminal care we reviewed: several dimensions of satisfaction were assessed including satisfaction with availability, communication, continuity, interpersonal care, involvement in treatment decisions, pain management, technical care, and general satisfaction.

Construction of Multiple-Item Scales

Well-designed multiple-item scales tend to produce greater variability (differences between respondents), and to be more reliable and valid then single-item measures (Ware, 1981). The opportunity to control for acquiescent response set, one of the most prevalent forms of response bias in satisfaction research, is an advantage of using multiple items (Ware, 1978). Multiple items are particularly necessary to distinguish between the different dimensions of satisfaction (Ware et al., 1976a, 1976b). Despite the advantages of multiple-item scales, few of the studies we reviewed used more than a single item for each dimension of satisfaction with terminal care. Future research needs to follow the example of multiple-item scales provided in the studies by Kane and colleagues (Kane et al., 1985; Wales et al., 1983) and McCusker (1984).

Reliability

A reliability coefficient provides a direct estimate of the proportion of the total variance in a measure that is true score variance (see Marquis & Marquis, 1977). For example, a reliability coefficient of 0.80 means that 80% of the variance in a measure is true score or reliable variance and 20% of the variance is error variance. Thus, the extent to which a measure reflects true score variance rather than error variance defines the reliability of that measure. For *group* comparisons, a reliability of at least 0.50 is suggested (Helmstadter, 1964). For decisions about *individual* patients, much more stringent criteria are necessary (e.g., above 0.90 has been suggested by Ware, 1984).

Two of the more common methods for estimating reliability are internal consistency and test-retest. Internal consistency reliability involves examination of the covariation among items within hypothesized scales. It is a practical measure of reliability because only a single administration of the scale is required. Internal consistency is not applicable to single-item measures, however. When estimates of the reliability of individual items are needed, test-retest studies are necessary. The test-retest methodology involves administration of the same measures at two different time points. Test-retest reliability estimates are prone to bias due to subject recall and/or actual change in the construct being assessed (Ware, 1984).

None of the studies we reviewed that employed single item measures reported test-retest reliability estimates. In fact, the studies reported by Barbarin and Chesler (1984), Wales et al. (1983), and McCusker (1984), were the only ones providing reliability estimates at all. An internal consistency of 0.77 was found for Barbarin and Chesler's global satisfaction index. Wales et al. (1983) reported test-retest coefficients ranging from 0.71 to 0.98 for satisfaction with interpersonal care, satisfaction with humaneness, satisfaction with technical care, and general satisfaction. McCusker (1984) found acceptable internal consistency estimates (reliability estimates for different samples are separated by commas) for measures of general satisfaction (0.75, 0.85, 0.87), satisfaction with continuity of care (0.50, 0.53), satisfaction with physician interpersonal care (0.69, 0.85, 0.90), satisfaction with involvement of patient/family in treatment decisions (0.65), and satisfaction with pain control (0.66). Measures of satisfaction with availability of care (0.40, 0.61, 0.59) and technical care (0.41, 0.77, 0.78) were not internally consistent in one of the three samples she studied.

In studies measuring patient satisfaction with medical care, reliability has traditionally been estimated using the patient as the unit of analysis. However, there is a growing interest in physician-level reliability estimation to prevent "unit of analysis" error.

A unit of analysis error can occur when there is a confounding relationship between the substantive questions of the study (e.g., provider-level differences) and the statistical analysis (e.g., patient-level differences) performed (Whiting-O'Keefe, Henke, & Simborg, 1984). For example, the unit of analysis issue may be raised with respect to analyses of the effect of physician characteristics (e.g., physician nonverbal communication skills, system of care characteristics) on patient satisfaction. Research on patient satisfaction with care for terminal illness needs to examine reliability at the unit of analysis that is of concern. Physician-level reliability is calculated by comparing the extent to which different patients concur in their satisfaction with the same physician. Preliminary analyses of our own data indicate that physician-level reliability for patient satisfaction ratings is substantially lower than patient-level reliability. These results suggest that individual patients are consistent across satisfaction items, but different patients express different degrees of satisfaction with the same physician.

Validity

Validity is the extent to which a measure reflects the true construct or behavior it was intended to measure. The validity of a patient satisfaction measure refers to how well the measure represents satisfaction with medical care. Different strategies are used to evaluate validity, but correlations between satisfaction measures and carefully selected criterion measures are frequently involved in this evaluation. These correlations are examined to see how well they correspond to what would be expected for valid measures.

Validity may be evaluated on the basis of a measure's correlation with a variety of external criteria. For example, the relationship between patient satisfaction and behavioral intentions (e.g., intention to return to the doctor) has been used as a validity variable in patient satisfaction research (Hays & Ware, forthcoming). This form of validity is referred to as criterion validity.

Two of the most commonly used validity criteria are convergent and discriminant validity. Convergent validity indicates that a measure correlates with other measures with which it *should* correlate; discriminant validity is supported if a measure is shown to be independent of other measures with which it *should not* correlate. The multitrait-multimethod (MTMM) approach to validity assessment (Campbell & Fiske, 1959) involves simultaneous consideration of two or more traits measured in two or more ways (methods), permitting a standardized methodology for the assessment of convergent and discriminant validity of patient satisfaction measures. For example, both a patient and a significant other might be asked to report the patient's satisfaction with technical care, interpersonal care, and access to care. The patient and the significant other represent different *methods* of assessment, and the dimensions of care (technical, interpersonal, and access) represent different constructs.[4]

MTMM studies of patient satisfaction are very rare. Satisfaction with medical care is usually measured by only one method, asking the respondent directly. The MTMM methodology is not applicable to studies with only one method, but multitrait scaling, a MTMM-like analytic strategy, can be employed if multiple traits of patient satisfaction are assessed (Ware et al., 1983). This analytic technique goes beyond traditional internal consistency reliability because it tests *item* discrimination across scales. Convergent validity is supported if an item correlates substantially with the patient satisfaction scale it is designed to represent. Discriminant validity is supported if the item correlates more highly with the scale it was hypothesized to represent than with scales it was not supposed to represent. A good example of the use of multitrait scaling was provided in McCusker's (1984) study. Based on her assessment of convergent and discriminant validity, McCusker (1984) concluded that items measuring general satisfaction and satisfaction with physician availability performed adequately, but items in the three physician behavior scales (technical care, interpersonal care, and communication) could not be distinguished from one another.

Validity assessment of satisfaction measures used in studies of terminal care has been virtually nonexistent. McCusker's study (1984) was the only one to evaluate validity directly and Kane et al. (1985) adopted previously validated instruments. Given the basic importance of validity in scale evaluation, this deficiency in studies of satisfaction with care for the terminally ill is more in need of further attention than any of the other issues addressed in this paper.

SUMMARY

The importance of patient and family satisfaction with medical care during the terminal phase of life is underscored by increasing concerns about the quality of life of the terminally ill. Surveys of patient satisfaction with medical care have burgeoned in recent years. Similarly, a plethora of articles on death and dying have appeared. But, only a half-dozen studies of satisfaction with medical care among dying patients and their families could be located in the published literature.

Empirical studies of patient satisfaction have tended to be conducted without an explicit conceptual framework. In this paper, we have presented our social-psychological theory of patient satisfaction. The theory was used as a basis for understanding different approaches to patient satisfaction assessment and issues of concern for future research.

The significance of patient satisfaction as an outcome of medical care for the terminally ill demands the use of state-of-the art measures. Research on patient and family satisfaction with care for the terminally ill was examined in terms of data gathering medium (e.g., self-administered questionnaires, face to face interviews), patient satisfaction item structure (item stems and response options), dimensions of satisfaction (e.g., satisfaction with interpersonal care, satisfaction with technical care), construction of multiple-item scales, and reliability and validity of the measures.

Fundamental issues of reliability and validity were not addressed by the authors in the majority of studies we reviewed. Two exceptional studies were noted. Kane et al. (1985) adopted instruments that have been validated in other settings and that satisfy standard criteria for acceptability. In addition, the study by McCusker (1984) is distinguished by its pioneering work. The Kane et al. (1985) and McCusker (1984) studies provide the foundation upon which the state-of-the-art of assessing patient satisfaction with terminal illness can proceed.

ENDNOTES

1. The closer the correspondence between the components of the theory in terms of action, target at which the action is directed, the context in which it occurs, and time, the stronger the relationship between these components (Ajzen & Fishbein, 1980).

2. In a review of the literature, Torrens (1985) stated that no difference in patient satisfaction between hospice and conventional care patients was found in the National Hospice Study. The National Hospice Study was not included in our review, because we were unable to obtain documentation of satisfaction assessment in the study.

3. Ideally, values or perceived importance ratings would be combined with corresponding beliefs for the estimation of satisfaction. However, assessment of values as well as beliefs increases respondent burden considerably and may not have a significant effect on measured satisfaction because medical care values are highly interrelated (see e.g., Ware, Snyder, & Wright, 1976a, 1976b).

4. Ware et al. (1976b) provided four MTMM matrices that contained correlations of the Patient Satisfaction Questionnaire (PSQ) and global scales with satisfaction assessed by other methods (including a satisfaction continuum, "Very Satisfied" to "Very Dissatisfied"). Results from analyses of these matrices tended to support the convergent and discriminant validity of the PSQ measures. For example, we analyzed a matrix of correlations of PSQ Form II scales from one of the field tests using a recently developed computer program (Hays, in press; Hays & Hayashi, in press) and found that the average convergent validity correlation was 0.50 and that the majority of the discriminant validity comparisons were statistically significant in the hypothesized direction.

REFERENCES

Ajzen, I., & Fishbein, M. (1980). *Understanding attitudes and predicting social behavior.* Englewood Cliffs, New Jersey: Prentice-Hall.

Aroskar, M. A. (1985). Access to hospice: Ethical dimensions. *Nursing Clinics of North America, 20,* 299–309.

Bagozzi, R. P., & Burnkrant, R. E. (1985). Attitude organization and the attitude-behavior relation: A reply to Dillon and Kumar. *Journal of Personality and Social Psychology, 49,* 47–57.

Barbarin, O. A., & Chesler, M. A. (1984). Relationships with the medical staff and aspects of satisfaction with care expressed by parents of children with cancer. *Journal of Community Health, 9,* 302–313.

Barzelai, L. P. (1981). Evaluation of a home based hospice. *Journal of Family Practice, 12,* 241–245.

Bass, D. M. (1985). The hospice ideology and success of hospice care. *Research on Aging, 7,* 307–327.

Bollen, K. A., & Barb, K. H. (1981). Pearson's R and coarsely categorized measures. *American Sociological Review, 46,* 232–239.

Campbell, D. T., & Fiske, D. W. (1959). Convergent and discriminant validation by the multitrait-multimethod matrix. *Psychological Bulletin, 56,* 81–105.

Creek, L. V. (1982). A homecare hospice profile: Description, evaluation, and cost analysis. *Journal of Family Practice, 14,* 53–58.

Davies, A. R., & Ware, J. E. (1981). Measuring patient satisfaction with dental care. *Social Science and Medicine, 15A,* 751–760.

Davies, A. R., & Ware, J. E. (1982). *Development of a dental satisfaction questionnaire for the health insurance experiment.* Santa Monica, CA: The Rand Corporation, R-2712-HHS.

Dillman, D. A. (1978). *Mail and telephone surveys: The total design method.* New York: Wiley & Sons.

Dillon, W. R., & Kumar, A. (1985). Attitude organization and the attitude-behavior relation: A critique of Bagozzi and Burnkrant's reanalysis of Fishbein and Ajzen. *Journal of Personality and Social Psychology, 49,* 33–46.

Edwardson, S. R. (1985). Physician acceptance of home care for terminally ill children. *Health Services Research, 20,* 83–101.

Franco, V. W. (1985). The hospice: Humane care for the dying. *Journal of Religion and Health, 24,* 79–89.

Fulton, R. (1977). *Death, grief and bereavement. A bibliography: 1845–1975.* New York: Arno Press.

Hannon, E. L., & O'Donnell, J. F. (1984). An evaluation of hospices in the New York State hospice demonstration program. *Inquiry, 21,* 338–348.

Hays, R. (1985). An integrated value-expectancy theory of alcohol and other drug use. *British Journal of Addiction, 80,* 379–384.

Hays, R. (in press). MTMM.BAS: A program for analyzing multitrait-multimethod matrices. *Bulletin of the Society of Psychologists in Addictive Behaviors.*

Hays, R., & Hayashi, T. (in press). MTMM.EXE: A program for analyzing multitrait-multimethod matrices. *Applied Psychological Measurement.*

Hays, R., & Ware, J. E. (forthcoming). Short measures of patient satisfaction with specific medical encounters: A methodological comparison.

Helmstadter, G. C. (1964). *Principles of psychological measurement.* New York: Appleton-Century-Crofts.

Johnson, D. R., & Creech, J. L. (1983). Ordinal measures in multiple indicator models: A simulation study of categorization error. *American Sociological Review, 48,* 398–407.

Johnson, W. L., & Dixon, P. N. (1984). Response alternatives in Likert scaling. *Educational and Psychological Measurement, 44,* 563–567.

Kane, R. L., Klein, S. J., Bernstein, L., Rothenberg, R., & Wales, J. (1985). Hospice role in alleviating the emotional stress of terminal patients and their families. *Medical Care, 23,* 189–197.

Kastenbaum, R. (1979). "Healthy dying": A paradoxical quest continues. *Journal of Social Issues, 35,* 185–206.

Linder-Pelz, S. (1982). Toward a theory of patient satisfaction. *Social Science and Medicine, 16,* 577–582.

Lissitz, R. W., & Green, S. B. (1975). Effect of the number of scale points on reliability: A Monte Carlo approach. *Journal of Applied Psychology, 60,* 10–13.

Marquis, M. S., & Marquis, K. H. (1977). *Survey measurement design and evaluation using reliability theory.* Santa Monica, CA: The Rand Corporation (R-2088-HEW).

McCusker, J. (1984). Development of scales to measure satisfaction and preferences regarding long-term and terminal care. *Medical Care, 22,* 476–493.

Mor, V., & Kidder, D. (1985). Cost savings in hospices: Final results of the National hospice study. *Health Services Research, 20,* 407–422.

National Study Of Medical Care Outcomes. (1985). *National Study of Medical Care Outcomes Project Overview.* Santa Monica, CA: The Rand Corporation.

Paradis, L. F. (1984). Hospice program integration: An issue for policymakers. *Death Education, 8,* 383–398.

Pascoe, G. C. (1983). Patient satisfaction in primary health care: A literature review and analysis. *Evaluation And Program Planning, 6,* 185–210.

Rainey, L. C., Crane, L. A., Breslow, D. M., & Ganz, S. A. (1984). Cancer patients' attitudes toward hospice services. *Cancer: A Cancer Journal for Clinicians, 34,* 191–201.

Ramsay, J. O. (1973). The effect of number of categories in rating scales on precision of estimation of scale values. *Psychometrika, 38,* 513–532.

Risser, N. L. (1975). Development of an instrument to measure patient satisfaction with nurses and nursing care in primary care settings. *Nursing Research, 24,* 45–52.

Rosenberg, M. J., & Hovland, C. I. (1960). Cognitive, affective, and behavioral components of attitudes. In C. I. Hovland & M. J. Rosenberg (Eds.), *Attitude organization and change* (pp. 1–14). New Haven, Connecticut: Yale University Press.

Smith, S. A. (1984). The hospice concept as an alternative approach to management of terminal patients. *Pennsylvania Nurse, 39,* 8–9.

Torrens, P. R. (1985). Hospice care: What have we learned? *Annual Review of Public Health, 6,* 65–83.

VandenBos, G. R., DeLeon, P. H., & Pallak, M. S. (1982). An alternative to traditional medical care for the terminally ill: Humanitarian, policy, and political issues in hospice care. *American Psychologist, 37,* 1245–1248.

Wales, J., Kane, R., Robbins, S., Bernstein, L., & Krasnow, R. (1983). UCLA hospice evaluation study: Methodology and instrumentation. *Medical Care, 21,* 734–744.

Ware, J. E. (1978). Effects of acquiescent response set on patient satisfaction ratings. *Medical Care, 16,* 327–336.

Ware, J. E. (1981). How to survey patient satisfaction. *Drug Intelligence and Clinical Pharmacy, 15,* 892–899.

Ware, J. E. (1984). Methodological considerations in the selection of health status assessment procedures. In N.K. Wenger, M.E. Mattson, K. Furberg, & J. Elinson (Eds.), *Assessment of quality of life in clinical trials of cardiovascular disease* (pp. 87–111). New York: Le Jacq Publishers.

Ware, J. E., Davies-Avery, A., & Stewart, A. L. (1978). The measurement and meaning of patient satisfaction. *Health and Medical Services Review, 1,* 1–15.

Ware, J. E., Johnston, S. A., Davies-Avery, A., & Brook, R. H. (1979). *Conceptualization and measurement of health for adults in the health insurance study, Vol. 3: Mental Health.* Santa Monica, CA: The Rand Corporation, R-1987/3-HEW.

Ware, J. E., Snyder, M. K., & Wright, W. R. (1976a). *Development and validation of scales to measure patient satisfaction with health care services: Volume I of a final report. Part A: Review of literature, overview of methods, and results regarding construction of scales.* (NTIS Publication No. PB 288-329). Springfield, VA: National Technical Information Service.

Ware, J. E., Snyder, M. K., & Wright, W. R. (1976b). *Development and validation of scales to measure patient satisfaction with health care services: Volume I of a final report. Part B: Results regarding scales constructed from the patient satisfaction questionnaire and measures of other health care perceptions.* (NTIS Publication NO. PB 288-330). Springfield, VA: National Technical Information Service.

Ware, J. E., Snyder, M. K., Wright W. R., & Davies, A. R. (1983). Defining and measuring patient satisfaction with medical care. *Evaluation and Program Planning, 6,* 247–263.

Whiting-O'Keefe, Q. E., Henke, C., & Simborg, D. W. (1984). Choosing the correct unit of analysis in medical care experiments. *Medical Care, 22,* 1101–1114.